Contents

List of Figures v

List of Tables vii

About the Authors xi

Preface xiii

Chapter 1. An Introduction to Cardiovascular Services 1

Chapter 2. Dimensions of Change
in the Cardiovascular Market 19

Chapter 3. Local Market Assessment 51

Chapter 4. Program Strategy Development 81

Chapter 5. Program Management 105

Chapter 6. Financial Management 129

Chapter 7. Cardiovascular Surgery Program Planning 167

Chapter 8. Strategic Marketing Plan 187

Chapter 9. Diagnostic and Therapeutic Cardiovascular
Technology 203

Chapter 10. Cardiovascular Services Facilities and Equipment 229

Chapter 11. Case Studies 245

Chapter 12. Cardiovascular Institute Development 263

Appendix A. Cardiovascular Surgery and Invasive Cardiology
Services Business Plan 275

Appendix B. Cardiovascular Services Strategic Business
            Plan Outline 277

Appendix C. Cardiovascular Services Implementation
            Questionnaire 281

Appendix D. Cardiovascular Services Strategic Marketing
            Plan Outline 287

Appendix E. Cardiovascular Institute Business
            Plan Outline 289

Glossary 295

Successful Management Strategies in Cardiovascular Services

Philip L. Ronning
John W. Meyer
Charles W. Franc

AHA books are published by American Hospital Publishing, Inc.,
an American Hospital Association company

The views expressed in this publication are strictly those of the authors and do not necessarily represent official positions of the American Hospital Association.

Library of Congress Cataloging-in-Publication Data

Ronning, Philip L.
   Successful management strategies in cardiovascular services /
Philip L. Ronning, John W. Meyer, Charles W. Franc.
      p.   cm.
   Includes bibliographical references.
   ISBN 1-55648-083-0 (pbk.)
   1. Hospitals — Cardiovascular services — Management.   I. Meyer, John W.,
1947-   .   II. Franc, Charles W.   III. Title.
   [DNLM: 1. Cardiovascular Diseases — prevention & control.   WG 100
R773s]
   RA975.5.C3R66   1992
   362.1'961'0068 — dc20
   DNLM/DLC
   for Library of Congress   91-47042
                                                                              CIP

Catalog no. 067300

© 1992 by American Hospital Publishing, Inc.,
an American Hospital Association company

Printed in the USA

AHA is a service mark of the American Hospital Association used under license by American Hospital Publishing, Inc.

Text set in English Times
3M — 3/92 — 0313

Marlene Chamberlain, Project Editor
Linda Conheady, Manuscript Editor
Nancy Charpentier, Editorial Assistant
Marcia Bottoms, Managing Editor
Peggy DuMais, Production Coordinator
Susan Edge-Gumbel, Designer
Brian Schenk, Books Division Director

List of Figures

Figure 1-1. Selected 1991 Data on Cardiovascular Disease 3

Figure 1-2. Diagram of the Heart 8

Figure 2-1. Hospital Reimbursement Trends 35

Figure 2-2. The Product Life Cycle 41

Figure 2-3. Strategic Program Elements 44

Figure 3-1. CV Program Assessment and Strategic Planning
Process 53

Figure 3-2. Forces That Affect Competition and Strategy 75

Figure 4-1. The Value Chain 83

Figure 4-2. Strategy Formulation Process 85

Figure 4-3. Cardiovascular Services: Strategic Action Matrix 88

Figure 4-4. Scenario One: SWOT Analysis and Critical Success
Factors (Regional Perspective) 90

Figure 4-5. Cardiovascular Services: Sample Guiding Principles 91

Figure 4-6. Cardiovascular Program Structural Variables Analysis
(Based on Interview Results) 94

Figure 4-7. Cardiovascular Program Organizational Elements
(Based on Interview Results) 96

Figure 7-1. Schematic of CVS Development Program 174

Figure 7-2. CVS Development Program Implementation Task
Force Schedule.................................176

Figure 7-3. CVS Development Program Task Force
Organization Worksheet..........................179

Figure 7-4. Task Force and Subcommittee Responsibility
Checklist......................................180

Figure 7-5. CVS Development Program Implementation
Schedule/Timetable.............................183

Figure 8-1. Strategic Marketing Planning Process...............189

Figure 8-2. Differentiation Strategies: Cardiovascular Services....191

Figure 8-3. Typical Data Requirements for a Cardiovascular
Marketing Plan.................................192

Figure 8-4. Major Market Segments and Submarkets............194

Figure 8-5. Major Markets and Identification of Program
Selection Criteria...............................195

Figure 8-6. Sample Strategies and Tactics for a Cardiovascular
Surgery Program...............................199

Figure 10-1. Schematic Design for Cardiac Catheterization
Laboratory....................................234

Figure 10-2. Schematic Layout for a Dedicated Cardiovascular
Surgery Department............................236

Figure 10-3. Schematic Design for a Dedicated CSICU..........238

Figure 11-1. Whitney Hospital: Total Admissions to CSICU,
1983–1988.....................................257

Figure 12-1. Cardiovascular Institute:
Traditional Hospital Model......................264

Figure 12-2. Model for an Evolving Cardiovascular Institute......265

Figure 12-3. Heart Institute Development (Scenario Issues)........269

List of Tables

Table 1-1. Age-Adjusted Death Rates for Selected Causes of Death 4

Table 1-2. Death Rates for Diseases of the Heart 4

Table 1-3. Discharge Rates and Days of Care 4

Table 1-4. Cardiovascular Operations and Procedures 5

Table 1-5. Utilization Rates for Cardiovascular Procedures 5

Table 1-6. Utilization Rates for Total Cardiac Catheterization Procedures 6

Table 1-7. Utilization Rates for Diagnostic and Therapeutic Catheterization Procedures 6

Table 1-8. Utilization Rates for Cardiac Surgery Procedures 6

Table 2-1. U.S. Hospitals Providing Cardiac Catheterization and Cardiovascular Surgery 20

Table 2-2. U.S. Hospitals Providing Cardiac Catheterization and Cardiovascular Surgery by Region 22

Table 2-3. Distribution of Cardiovascular Programs by State: 1990 24

Table 2-4. Distribution of Selected Cardiovascular Programs by Region: 1990 25

Table 2-5. State Ranking by Population per Catheterization Laboratory: 1990 26

Table 2-6. State Ranking by Population per Cardiovascular
Surgery Program: 1990 27

Table 2-7. Comparison of Case Prices and Volume for Bypass
Procedure (DRG 107): California, 1988 30

Table 3-1. Demographic Analysis of Sample Hospital's
Service Area 60

Table 3-2. Market Share by Zip Code and Product Line,
Antelope Valley Market Area 62

Table 3-3. Sample Community Hospital Cardiovascular
Services Product Line Summary, Primary
Market Area: FY 1986 63

Table 3-4. Financial Class Utilization of Cardiovascular
Services by Zip Code and Product Line 64

Table 3-5. Sample Community Hospital Patients Discharged,
Age Distribution by Zip Code: 1988 67

Table 3-6. Sample Community Hospital Market Share
Summary: Top Four Market Share Positions by
Cardiovascular Services Product Line,
Primary Market Area 68

Table 3-7. Sample Community Hospital Cardiovascular
Services Use Rate Projections 69

Table 5-1. Cardiovascular Product Line Inventory 114

Table 6-1. Computer Model: Basic Assumptions 132

Table 6-2. Computer Model: Capital Cost Assumptions 134

Table 6-3. Computer Model: Income Statement 136

Table 6-4. Computer Model: Cash Flow, Distributions,
and Return on Investment 138

Table 6-5. Reimbursement by Payer Class 152

Table 6-6. Discharges, Average Charges, and LOS
for DRGs 104–107, 112, 124, 125:
HCFA CY 1987 (age 65+) 156

Table 6-7. Cardiovascular DRGs (Diseases/Disorders
of the Circulatory System) 161

Table 10-1. Sample Cardiovascular Services Space
Design Program 231

Table 10-2. Cardiovascular Surgery Department
Equipment List 240

Table 10-3. Cardiac Catheterization Laboratory
Equipment List 242

Table 10-4. Cardiovascular Surgery Intensive Care Unit 243

Table 11-1. General Medical Center, Cardiovascular Surgery
and PTCA: Initial Financial Results
of STP Protocol 251

Table 11-2. Results of Program Development Efforts 253

Table 12-1. Heart Institute Development Options 267

Table 12-2. Assumption Analysis 268

Table 12-3. Cardiovascular Institute: Projected Five-Year
Operating Budget 272

About the Authors

Philip L. Ronning has had extensive health care, hospital, and consulting experience in administration, finance, and strategy formation. Specifically, his consulting experience includes a position with the largest nonprofit hospital corporation in the United States, as well as being president of his own firm. Specializing in strategic planning, financial feasibility assessment, joint venture development, diversification planning, strategy formation, and physician practice management, he is uniquely qualified in the area of clinical program management.

Mr. Ronning earned a master's degree in hospital and health care administration from St. Louis University and is an Advanced Member of the Hospital Financial Management Association and a member of the American College of Healthcare Executives. He publishes and lectures extensively throughout the United States and serves on the American Hospital Association's Clinical Services and Technology Advisory Panel; he also provides consulting services for hospitals, physicians, medical groups, hospital systems, and emerging health care businesses.

John W. Meyer has more than 16 years of health care, hospital, and consulting experience. Specializing in strategic planning, marketing, and strategy development, he has considerable expertise in the areas of oncology and cardiovascular services. He has extensive experience as director of planning and director of marketing for community, tertiary, nonprofit, and proprietary hospitals in southern California.

Mr. Meyer earned a master's degree in hospital administration from the University of California at Berkeley and is a Fellow of the American College of Healthcare Executives. He has published and lectured extensively while providing consulting services for hospitals, physicians, medical groups, and emerging health care businesses.

Charles W. Franc has more than 14 years of health care, hospital, and consulting experience in administrative, technical, and clinical areas. Twelve years of his experience has been in cardiovascular medicine, most recently as director of cardiology for a large, urban, tertiary hospital in southern California. Focusing on the operational and management aspects of health care, he specializes in cardiovascular services and provides consulting services for hospitals, physicians, medical groups, and medical equipment manufacturers across the United States.

Preface

Cardiovascular disease is the leading cause of death in America, represents the largest source of nonobstetric hospital admissions, and accounts for the highest percentage of patient hospital days of stay.

As recently as 10 years ago, most major cardiac procedures were done only at tertiary centers that had open-heart surgery programs. By 1990, however, the number of hospitals offering cardiac catheterization services had grown by nearly 52 percent, and the number of hospitals offering cardiovascular surgery had grown by nearly 48 percent. This growth is due directly to the fact that use of diagnostic and therapeutic catheterization has grown faster than the population.

The revenue-generating potential of cardiovascular services is significant, to say the least. Furthermore, spin-off revenue — that income ascribed to patients who present with cardiovascular disease as a second or comorbid condition — is also a meaningful portion of overall hospital revenues.

These realities, combined with technological advancements (such as echocardiography and nuclear cardiography) that make cardiovascular services available on an outpatient basis, have opened the way for intense competition among providers. In addition, changing criteria for reimbursement and patient services contracts with managed care firms are forcing providers — already hard-pressed to control runaway health care costs — to be more competitive in the areas of cost and quality of service.

These trends are expected to shape the cardiovascular services market in the future:

- Major centers will lose market share.
- Prices for cardiovascular surgery will drop and then will stabilize.
- The number of cardiovascular programs will continue to grow.

- Technological innovation will continue.
- Reimbursement methods and mechanisms for hospitals and physicians will continue to change.

This book is intended as a resource to hospital executives, managers, and planners, as well as physicians interested in the planning and operations of cardiovascular programs. The scope of the book will allow seasoned managers to gain fresh perspectives and to challenge conventional assumptions about the evolving cardiovascular services market, provide basic information to those new to the field, and serve as a practical guide for hospitals that may be considering the addition of invasive cardiology and/or cardiovascular surgery services. The book will familiarize the reader with industry trends and developing technology and their effects on the hospitals and physicians in the market. It also will describe procedures for program planning, alternatives for organization, and a variety of operational issues related to implementing and managing successful cardiovascular programs. A working computer model is provided to help planners set up a long-term strategy for financial development and monitoring of a new or expanded cardiovascular program.

Six case studies give examples of strategies and tactics used by hospitals in different positions within their markets, showing the outcome for each.

The broad scope of the topic makes it necessary to cover a lot of ground while trying to observe space limitations. Therefore, certain subjects — promotional campaigns, patient education, outreach programs, clinical job descriptions, and the like — are treated only as they relate to unique aspects of cardiovascular programs.

This book builds on many of the concepts presented in our previous volume, *Developing Effective Invasive Cardiology Services,* written with Steven Lewis and published by the American Hospital Association. In both volumes, the state of California is used as an example because of the maturity of its market, the authors' familiarity with it, and the extensive nature of the data system operated by the California Office of Statewide Health Planning and Development.

Chapter 1

An Introduction
to Cardiovascular Services

As recently as 10 years ago, cardiovascular (CV) services were relatively uncommon in small community hospitals. Today, however, CV services rank consistently as the most strategically and financially important product line for U.S. hospitals, both large and small.

For readers who may be new to the field, this chapter provides background information on cardiovascular services as a product line in hospitals, including various dimensions of the field — demographics, range of diseases treated, range of professionals involved, and so forth. Specific topics include the following:

1. Demographic factors related to increased use of CV services (projected changes and trends will be explored in chapter 2)
2. Cardiovascular anatomy, physiology, and pathology
3. Clinical foundations of cardiovascular and circulatory disease, diagnosis, and treatment as applied to development, planning, and management for CV services
4. The practice of cardiovascular medicine and key physician practitioners
5. Organization of cardiovascular services in hospitals
6. The industrial principle of product line management as it relates to CV services

Several terms are used throughout the book to describe this product line. *Cardiovascular* and *cardiac* can be used interchangeably to refer to all heart services. *Cardiology* is a subspecialty within internal medicine, whereas *cardiovascular surgery* is a subspecialty of thoracic (chest) surgery. Note that, as a term describing a set of services, *cardiology* does not include the surgical aspects of cardiovascular services. Therefore, *cardiovascular services* will be used throughout this book to refer to all heart services (occasionally the acronym *CVS* or the term *CV services* is also used).

Increased Utilization of Cardiovascular Services in Hospitals

Cardiovascular services are among the most important and competitive service markets in health care. The growth of this market is a direct result of the fact that cardiac disease continues to affect more Americans than any other disease. The American Heart Association calculates that heart disease is the number one cause of death in the United States, claiming nearly a million lives in 1988, and that currently more than 68 million Americans suffer from some form of cardiovascular disease.[1] It is estimated that nearly half of all Americans will die of heart disease. Figure 1-1 highlights additional statistics that show the dimensions of cardiovascular disease in the United States. Table 1-1 shows the age-adjusted death rates per 100,000 persons for major causes of death over a five-year period. Note that although death rates are declining, the death rate from heart disease is still approximately 25 percent higher than the death rate from cancer (malignant neoplasms). The overall death rate from heart disease, when not adjusted for age, also continues to decline but remains significant (table 1-2).

As the leading cause of death in America, cardiovascular disease accounted for 45.3 percent of all deaths in 1988.[2] Furthermore, as documented in table 1-3, it is the primary source of nonobstetric hospital admissions and the principal diagnosis, accounting for the largest percentage of patient hospital days.[3] Cardiovascular treatments account for the largest single component of the health care dollar, estimated by the American Heart Association to be more than $100,000,000 in 1991.[4]

Of all CV procedures conducted from 1979 to 1987, the volume increased not only of cardiac catheterizations, but also of percutaneous transluminal coronary angioplasty (PTCA, described in chapter 2) and cardiovascular surgery (table 1-4). Table 1-5 presents the national rates for diagnostic cardiac catheterizations, coronary artery bypass grafts (CABGs), cardiac valve surgeries, PTCAs, and permanent pacemaker implants (PPIs). By expressing the rate of these procedures per 1,000 population per year, the table underscores the fact that utilization of these procedures is growing faster than the population. Therefore, the actual and potential size of the cardiovascular services market certainly warrants the attention of hospitals. In fact, purchasers of cardiovascular services form the largest of the health care services markets.

Although gross national data provide a useful overview, institutions must obtain and analyze statistics specific to their service area to plan for CV services that are market based. (Chapter 3 provides a detailed discussion of market assessment.) For example, the national utilization rates shown in tables 1-1 through 1-5 are then compared in tables 1-6, 1-7, and 1-8 with utilization rates in the state of California and in Los Angeles County, both high-volume areas for CV services and both mature markets with high levels of competition and physician saturation. Table 1-6 compares total national and regional cardiac catheterization rates. Table 1-7 compares diagnostic and therapeutic cardiac catheterization use rates for the nation and California. Table 1-8 extracts use rates for cardiovascular surgery.

The rates generally were higher in California and Los Angeles during the early 1980s but now are trending lower than the national rates. There are many reasons for this: relatively inaccurate national data bases; size of data base; opportunity for error; and rebound effect of pent-up demand for these services, a demand now being satisfied in suburban, semirural, and rural areas that previously lacked direct access to CV physician specialists. Whatever the cause, these differences underscore the need for access to local information and ability to compute these local rates on as recent a basis as possible.

Figure 1-1. Selected 1991 Data on Cardiovascular Disease

Coronary Disease
- 6,060,000 Americans have a history of heart attack, chest pain, or both (2.5%).
- 1,500,000 were estimated to have had heart attacks in 1991, 500,000 of whom died.

Chest Pain (Angina Pectoris)
- 3,040,000 Americans have experienced chest pain (1.2%).
- 300,000 new cases of angina occur each year according to the Framingham Heart Study.

High Blood Pressure (Hypertension)
- 61,870,000 Americans have high blood pressure (25.2%).
- 30,960 died in 1988 as a result of hypertension.
- 46.1% of hypertensives are unaware of their condition.

Congenital Heart Defects
- 5,600 deaths were attributed to congenital heart defects.
- 920,000 Americans have congenital heart defects (0.37%).
- 25,000 babies are born each year with heart defects.
- 35 types of congenital heart defects have been identified.

Heart Transplantation
- 1,676 transplants were performed in 1989.
- The average 30-day mortality rate is 9.7%.
- The 5-year survival rate is 81%.
- The 10-year survival rate is 73%.

Adapted from *1991 Heart and Stroke Facts,* American Heart Association, Dallas, TX, 1991.

Table 1-1. Age-Adjusted Death Rates for Selected Causes of Death: United States, 1983–1987 (per 100,000 population)

Cause of Death	1983	1984	1985	1986	1987
All causes	550.5	545.9	546.1	541.7	535.5
Diseases of the heart	188.8	183.6	180.5	175.0	169.6
Malignant neoplasms	132.6	133.5	133.6	133.2	132.9
Accidents and adverse effects	35.3	35.0	34.7	35.2	34.6
Cerebrovascular diseases	34.4	33.4	32.3	31.0	30.3
Chronic obstructive pulmonary disease	17.4	17.7	18.7	18.8	18.7
Pneumonia and influenza	11.8	12.2	13.4	13.5	13.1
Suicide	11.4	11.6	11.5	11.9	11.7
Diabetes mellitus	9.9	9.5	9.6	9.6	9.8
Chronic liver disease and cirrhosis	10.2	10.0	9.6	9.2	9.1
Homicide and legal intervention	8.6	8.4	8.3	9.0	8.6

Source: National Center for Health Statistics, *Health, United States, 1989*, Hyattsville, MD: Public Health Service, 1990.

Table 1-2. Death Rates for Diseases of the Heart (per 100,000 population)

	1982	1983	1984	1985	1986	1987
Death rate	326.0	329.2	323.5	323.0	317.5	312.4
Age-adjusted death rate	190.5	188.8	183.6	180.5	175.0	169.6

Source: National Center for Health Statistics, *Health, United States, 1989*, Hyattsville, MD: Public Health Service, 1990.

Table 1-3. Discharge Rates and Days of Care (per 1,000 population)

First-Listed Diagnosis	Number of Discharges				Days of Care			
	1980	1985	1987	1988	1980	1985	1987	1988
Females with delivery	14.7	14.1	14.0	13.4	55.5	46.1	42.8	39.2
Diseases of heart	13.1	13.7	13.8	13.2	123.5	98.4	94.5	92.2
Malignant neoplasms	7.6	7.4	7.1	6.2	90.5	65.2	60.8	57.6
Fracture, all sites	4.9	4.4	4.0	3.8	51.2	37.1	34.3	30.8
Pneumonia, all forms	3.5	3.6	3.7	3.6	27.7	26.5	27.7	28.5
Total	159.1	138.0	127.9	117.8	1,136.5	877.1	808.7	754.8

Source: National Center for Health Statistics, *Health, United States, 1989*, Hyattsville, MD: Public Health Service, 1990.

Table 1-4.   Cardiovascular Operations and Procedures: United States, 1979–1987 (estimate in thousands)

Procedure	1979	1980	1981	1982	1983	1984	1985	1986	1987
Valves	33	35	35	37	37	42	44	46	43
Coronary artery bypass grafts	114	137	159	170	191	202	230	284	332
Pacemaker insert, maintenance and removal	172	187	177	202	190	209	223	215	233
Cardiac catheterizations	299	348	414	471	508	570	681	775	866
Angioplasties	2	6	6	12	26	46	82	133	184
Other vascular and cardiac surgery[a]	625	739	850	946	1,023	1,100	1,207	1,370	1,493
Total procedures excluding hemodialysis	1,245	1,452	1,641	1,838	1,975	2,169	2,467	2,823	3,151
Total open-heart surgery[a]	166	195	217	239	266	310	372	478	581

[a]Includes 19,000 "other" open-heart surgeries in 1979; 23,000 in 1980 and 1981; 32,000 in 1982; 38,000 in 1983; 66,000 in 1984; 98,000 in 1985; 148,000 in 1986; and 206,000 in 1987.

Source: National Center for Health Statistics.

Table 1-5.   Utilization Rates for Cardiovascular Procedures: United States (per 1,000 population)

Year	Dx Caths	CABGs	Valves	PTCAs	All PPIs
1982	2.03	0.73	0.16	0.05	0.87
1983	2.17	0.82	0.16	0.11	0.81
1984	2.41	0.85	0.18	0.19	0.88
1985	2.85	0.96	0.18	0.34	0.93
1986	3.23	1.18	0.19	0.55	0.90
1987	3.56	1.36	0.18	0.76	0.96

Abbreviations: Dx Caths, diagnostic cardiac catheterizations; CABGs, coronary artery bypass grafts; valves, cardiac valve surgeries; PTCAs, percutaneous transluminal coronary angioplasties; PPIs, permanent pacemaker insertions.

Sources: National Center for Health Statistics; Statistical Abstract of the United States, 1989, Hyattsville, MD, 1990.

Table 1-6. Utilization Rates for Total Cardiac Catheterization Procedures (per 1,000 population)

Year	United States	California	Los Angeles
1983	2.28	2.93	3.13
1984	2.60	3.32	3.43
1985	3.19	3.65	3.68
1986	3.78	4.25	4.30
1987	4.32	4.90	5.00
1988	Unavailable	5.37	5.17

Sources: California Office of Statewide Health Planning and Development; National Center for Health Statistics, 1989.

Table 1-7. Utilization Rates for Diagnostic and Therapeutic Catheterization Procedures (per 1,000 population)

Year	Diagnostic			Therapeutic		
	United States	California	Los Angeles	United States	California	Los Angeles
1983	2.17	2.78	2.99	0.11	0.15	0.14
1984	2.41	2.99	3.09	0.19	0.33	0.34
1985	2.85	3.09	3.15	0.34	0.56	0.53
1986	3.23	3.51	3.60	0.55	0.74	0.70
1987	3.56	3.95	4.09	0.76	0.95	0.91
1988	Unavailable	4.28	4.12	Unavailable	1.09	1.05

Sources: California Office of Statewide Health Planning and Development; National Center for Health Statistics.

Table 1-8. Utilization Rates for Cardiac Surgery Procedures (per 1,000 population)

Year	United States	California	Los Angeles
1983	0.98	0.99	1.05
1984	1.03	0.92	0.94
1985	1.14	0.91	0.93
1986	1.37	0.97	0.98
1987	1.54	1.02	1.00
1988	Unavailable	1.10	1.06

Note: Total U.S. rate is total of CABG and valve surgery from table 1-5.

Sources: California Office for Statewide Health Planning and Development; National Center of Health Statistics.

The broad dimension of the health problem, coupled with the rapid pace of technological advancements in the diagnosis and treatment of cardiac disease in recent years, makes cardiovascular services one of the most intensely competitive health care markets. For example:

- Technological progress has helped lower the barriers of cost and complexity, with the result that more providers compete for market share.
- This competition is fueled by the fact that reimbursement from managed care firms and third-party administrators remains comparatively equitable.
- The number of cardiovascular surgery programs in community hospitals has increased dramatically. Whereas several years ago only tertiary centers with open-heart surgery programs had cardiology departments, today almost all hospitals have some type of cardiology department.
- Physicians have become a significant competitive force in the market for diagnostic services, particularly in *echocardiography* (ultrasound).
- The technological improvements that allow a cardiac catheterization laboratory to operate as an outpatient facility with no hospital affiliation have also resulted in competition from solo practitioners and physician group practices for a service traditionally provided by hospitals.

This diffusion of cardiovascular technology is not the result of a single breakthrough but rather a result of increased expertise among those involved at all levels of CV patient care. The result is a market that is competitive and yet still attractive for hospitals.

The next two sections provide, respectively, a briefing on cardiovascular anatomy for nonclinicians and a look at the major cardiac diseases. Both topics are suggestive of the range of service options.

Anatomy and Physiology of the Heart

The heart is a muscular organ composed of four distinct chambers, which serve as collection areas for blood during the phases of cardiac activity. The four chambers are paired on separate sides of the heart—the *right-sided* and *left-sided* chambers. The right-sided chambers include the *right atrium* and the *right ventricle;* the left-sided chambers are the *left atrium* and the *left ventricle.* (See figure 1-2.) In a normal heart, the left and right sides are separated by an inner wall, the *septum,* which in turn has two major sections, the *interatrial septum* and the *interventricular septum.* The two chambers of each side of the heart are separated by a cardiac valve. These valves, which separate the *atria* (plural of *atrium*) from the ventricles, are known

Figure 1-2. Diagram of the Heart

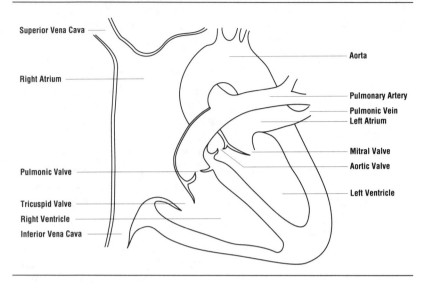

Superior Vena Cava

Right Atrium

Aorta

Pulmonary Artery

Pulmonic Vein

Left Atrium

Mitral Valve

Aortic Valve

Pulmonic Valve

Left Ventricle

Tricuspid Valve

Right Ventricle

Inferior Vena Cava

as *atrioventricular valves.* The valve between the right atrium and the right ventricle is called the *tricuspid valve* because of its three leaflets (or cusps). The valve between the left atrium and the left ventricle is the *mitral valve,* which was formerly called the bicuspid valve.

Two more cardiac valves, known as *semilunar valves,* are found at the exit regions of each ventricle. The right ventricle exit valve is the *pulmonic* (or pulmonary) *valve;* it adjoins the *pulmonary artery.* The valve at the left ventricle exit is the *aortic valve,* positioned between the left ventricle and the aorta.

The heart's right-sided and left-sided chambers, along with their associated structures, perform nearly identical functions but are responsible for the circulation of the blood in different phases. The chambers on the right side of the heart provide the pumping activity to circulate blood to and through the lungs. The chambers on the left side pump oxygenated blood from the lungs through the body and tissues. Because of the significant difference in the areas to which the right and left ventricles pump their blood volume, a noticeably different pressure must be generated by each ventricle. Because the left ventricle must force blood through a much greater volume of tissue, it must generate more pressure than the right ventricle. Typically, a healthy left ventricle will generate a peak pressure of 120 mm Hg (millimeters of mercury), with the right ventricle averaging a 25–30 mm Hg peak pressure. Because the left ventricle must generate greater pressure, the left ventricular muscle mass must exceed that of the right ventricle. More muscle tissue translates into the need for a larger blood supply, which in turn requires a greater number of coronary arteries to supply the larger volume of blood. Because the left ventricle is supplied by more blood vessels than the right ventricle and must work harder to generate greater pressure, its surrounding muscle tissue (the *myocardium*) is vastly more susceptible to heart attack from coronary artery obstructions.

The following description may help the reader visualize the path the blood follows as it flows through the heart and vasculature. First, blood returning from the body—that is, blood whose oxygen has been used by the body's tissues—is called venous blood. The returning venous blood collects in the right atrium. While the right atrium collects venous blood, the right ventricle contracts and ejects its blood volume through the pulmonic valve into the pulmonary artery. As the right ventricle begins to relax from its contracted state, a pressure differential is created across the tricuspid valve between the right atrium and right ventricle. As it relaxes, the right ventricle is at a lower pressure than the blood collected in the right atrium. This pressure differential causes the blood in the right atrium to force open the tricuspid valve and begin to flow into the relaxing right ventricle.

Shortly after this flow begins, an electrical signal is generated by the heart's natural pacemaker, which is known as the *sinoatrial (SA) node*. The SA node is located in the right atrium. This electrical signal is conducted through the muscle tissue of both the right and left atria, causing the tissue to begin contracting. At this time, the tissue of the right ventricle is almost fully relaxed (the left ventricle is simultaneously completing its relaxation as well). The right atrium has begun contracting, forcing more blood into the right ventricle through the tricuspid valve (again, this process is being mirrored by the chambers on the left side). As the right atrium completes its contraction and begins to relax, a pressure differential is created in reverse from that previously described. Now the lower pressure is in the atrium, and as it continues to relax further, blood attempts to flow back into the atrium. This slight reversal of blood flow "catches" on the billowy leaflets of the tricuspid valve (this is occurring in the chambers on the left side nearly simultaneously with the mitral valve), causing the valve to close and stop the reversed blood flow.

At this point, the electrical signal generated in the SA node has reached the *atrioventricular (AV) node* located between the atria and ventricles. After detaining this signal briefly to allow the mechanical contraction of the atria to occur, the AV node releases its signal to the ventricular muscle tissue. The right ventricle (as well as the left) has completed its filling process, the tricuspid valve (and the mitral valve) has closed, the atria have begun to relax (which causes them to begin filling from "above" as the reversed blood flow from the ventricles has been stopped by the tricuspid and mitral valves), and the electrical signal from the AV node causes the ventricles to begin contracting. With the tricuspid and mitral valves closed, this ventricular contraction causes the blood volume in the right ventricle to be forced through the pulmonic valve into the pulmonary artery.

Meanwhile, the blood under pressure from the right ventricle continues to be forced through the pulmonary artery and smaller branch arteries into the lungs, where it undergoes a process that gives up carbon dioxide, a waste-product gas, from the body's tissues and collects oxygen from the air in the lungs. This process occurs in very small capillary blood vessels within the lungs. The oxygen-rich blood then begins to drain from the lungs through a series of enlarging branch vessels known as *pulmonic veins.* These vessels eventually connect with the four main pulmonary veins that connect directly with the left atrium.

Next, the oxygen-carrying blood fills the left atrium as it undergoes its relaxation and filling stage. The left atrium fills with blood, the left ventricle begins to relax after contracting (simultaneously with the right ventricle), the mitral valve between the left atrium and ventricle is forced open because of the pressure differential across it, and blood begins to flow into the left ventricle from the left atrium. The electrical signal from the SA node reaches the left atrium and causes it to contract with the right atrium, forcing blood into the left ventricle. As the left atrium begins to relax, the pressure differential is reversed across the mitral valve, which causes a reversal of blood flow. This reversed blood flow causes the mitral valve leaflets to close; the left atrium continues to fill from the pulmonic veins while the electrical signal has reached the AV node and is subsequently released and sent to the left ventricle, causing it to contract.

The left ventricle contracts, forcing its blood volume through the aortic valve into the *aorta* (the body's main artery). The repeated contraction of the left ventricle and ejection of blood volume create the body's blood pressure and force the oxygen-enriched blood supply through the body's tissues. The oxygen-carrying blood is received by cells throughout the body, the oxygen is utilized, and carbon dioxide as a by-product of cellular metabolism is produced and then carried away by the blood. This "used" blood, or venous blood, begins to flow back toward the heart to become reoxygenated. The venous blood flows through a series of enlarging vessels (veins) until it eventually reaches the largest veins, the *superior vena cava* and *inferior vena cava.* These venae cavae are attached directly to the right atrium, and the venous blood now reenters the right atrium to begin the process again. In a normal heart, this fill–contract–eject–refill cycle occurs in less than one second.

The heart, then, is an intricate, highly complex, and active organ. Any number of diseases can endanger, interrupt, or even halt its functions.

Diseases of the Heart and Circulatory System

As indicated by figure 1-1, the significance of cardiovascular disease and its impact on hospitals cannot be overestimated. Heart disease, or abnormal cardiac anatomy (pathology), can be divided into two distinct groupings. The first includes diseases present at birth, referred to as *congenital cardiac diseases*. A congenital pathology generally results in abnormal cardiac structural development. These types of abnormalities can vary from mild to fatal in their effects on a patient's condition. Many forms of congenital heart disease are progressive in their severity and symptoms, whereas others can hold steady for years. The most common congenital cardiac diseases include holes in the heart wall, valve defects, abnormal heart size, malposition of the heart, or transposition of the great vessels.

The second and much more common type of cardiac disease includes the *acquired diseases of the heart.* This group is dominated by *coronary artery disease,* a condition caused primarily by the development of obstructive lesions (atherosclerotic plaque) within the arteries that supply the blood to the myocardium. Usually these obstructions to blood flow develop over time, and as the lesion (or lesions) continues to enlarge, it could restrict blood flow to the point where the myocardial region supplied by the affected artery receives blood volume inadequate to perform properly. This deficiency reduces contraction capabilities or, in the case of complete obstruction, causes death of that area of muscle tissue. Coronary artery disease varies widely in its effects on individuals, with the most severe effect being a heart attack *(myocardial infarction)* that proves fatal.

Other acquired diseases of the heart include *calcific valvular heart disease* (the accumulation of calcium deposits on a cardiac valve or valves); *infective and infiltrative diseases* (abnormalities of the cardiac conduction system); and *cardiomyopathy* (disease of the heart muscle) of several origins. Side effects of other diseases, such as diabetes and long-standing hypertension, also are evidenced frequently in their influence on the heart and its structures.

Professional intervention in CV disease typically begins with a diagnosis of cardiovascular disease made by a primary physician. Once dysfunction is diagnosed, a referral is made to a cardiologist, who obtains a history and performs a physical examination. In general, the diagnostic process involves a series of increasingly sophisticated noninvasive examinations, which may include an EKG (electrocardiograph), a stress EKG, a Holter monitor, or one of a variety of echocardiographic exams. As a rule, these studies are performed in the cardiologist's office or in a hospital cardiology department.

If a combination of patient risk factors, the physical examination, and the results of these noninvasive procedures indicates probability or existence of heart disease, a more advanced examination may be recommended, for example, a nuclear cardiographic examination, an advanced echocardiographic procedure, or a cardiac catheterization (an invasive procedure).

Based on results of these advanced cardiac examinations, a decision will be made regarding the patient's course of treatment. Treatment may include an interventional cardiac catheterization procedure, cardiovascular surgery, or medical management of the patient by the cardiologist.

The Practice of Cardiovascular Medicine

Medical doctors are divided into two basic groups: physicians and surgeons. In medical school, all doctors are provided with the same basic training. Upon completing their fourth year of medical school, they enter the first year of residency (formerly internship). Upon completing the one-year residency, doctors are considered either general or family practitioners, capable of performing an array of medical tasks. Doctors who choose further training will elect to enter either general internal medicine or general surgery. After another year's training and residency, they become general internists or general surgeons. Further training will qualify them to enter a *specialty*.

The Specialty of Cardiology

Cardiology is a specialty of internal medicine and typically requires a doctor to undergo two years of fellowship training to become a general cardiologist. An additional year or two of training qualifies the cardiologist to perform cardiac catheterizations, a procedure considered to be *invasive* cardiology because devices are inserted into the patient's body. A general cardiologist practices *noninvasive* cardiology if he or she performs noncatheterization procedures. Upon completing an additional year of fellowship training, a cardiologist is qualified to perform angioplasties or percutaneous transluminal coronary angioplasties (PTCAs), which are considered to be procedures of *interventional* cardiology. No special designation currently describes cardiologists who perform other interventional techniques, such as laser procedures and arthrectomies. Interventional cardiologists are, by definition, invasive cardiologists; however, not all invasive cardiologists are interventional cardiologists.

A cardiologist can also earn the designation of pediatric cardiologist, one whose work focuses on the younger (usually under age 17) cardiac patient who has congenital or birth-related disorders. Training in pediatric cardiology involves some pediatrics but is basically an area of interest and expertise acquired during the course of cardiology training. A pediatric cardiologist generally practices invasive cardiology because the cardiac catheterization laboratory is such a critical tool in the diagnosis of congenital anomalies.

A final specialty involves the diagnosis and treatment of cardiac conduction disorders, or *electrophysiology*.

Cardiovascular Surgery

Surgeons entering the cardiovascular field (specializing in blood vessels and circulatory conduction) must first become vascular surgeons (through additional fellowship), then thoracic surgeons, and, finally, cardiac surgeons. Therefore cardiac surgeons are referred to as cardiothoracic or cardiovascular surgeons. Pediatric cardiovascular surgeons require no special or extra training but generally demonstrate a slightly different set of skills.

Cardiologists refer many cases to cardiovascular surgeons, who perform invasive and interventional procedures that involve open-heart surgery (opening the chest cavity), bypass surgery (stopping the heart's activity during the procedure), or both. Open-heart procedures include pacemaker implantation, ablation, CABG, and heart transplants, among others. Bypass procedures — such as CABG or valve repair/replacement — involve temporarily replacing the heart's pumping action by means of a heart–lung machine. These and other cardiovascular therapies will be described in further detail in chapter 9.

Other Cardiovascular Specialties

Other physician participants on the cardiovascular team include the cardiac anesthesiologist, the physician responsible for administering local or general anesthesia and monitoring patient viability during a cardiac procedure. Cardiac anesthesiologists must have special training and experience, but generally a separate fellowship is not required. A cardiac anesthesiologist may be assisted by a nurse anesthetist, but a nurse anesthetist may not administer anesthesia without supervision.

Pulmonologists (internal medicine subspecialists) historically have not been trained specifically for cardiovascular work. Recently, however, certain pulmonologists, called *intensivists,* have focused more on the care of the critically ill. Intensivists can play a critical role in speeding the recovery of the postoperative cardiovascular patient.

Many other physicians are essential members of the cardiovascular team, but those described here are the key participants in patient care.

Organization of Cardiovascular Services in Hospitals

Cardiovascular surgery and cardiology are comparatively new medical specialties, neither having gained significant ground until the 1960s. At that time, cardiovascular surgery grew around a small number of university or community hospitals that, due to the presence of cardiology programs, were transformed into tertiary hospitals.

Cardiologists, invasive cardiologists in particular, practiced almost exclusively at these large centers because at the time and in most sections of the country cardiac catheterization could be performed only in hospitals that had open-heart surgery facilities. As more cardiologists were trained, they too located their practices near catheterization laboratories.

The large cardiac centers and tertiary hospitals also had departments that were organized to oversee the operation of noninvasive cardiovascular services. Often, the volume of cardiac patients was sufficient to warrant staff dedicated to the performing electrocardiography and other noninvasive diagnostic tests.

Generally, the catheterization laboratory and the noninvasive cardiology functions were combined into a single department under the supervision of a manager or director. The typical community hospital without cardiovascular surgery had neither cardiologists nor a dedicated department of cardiology. Initially, electrocardiograms (ECGs or EKGs) were performed by personnel from the clinical laboratory department, a practice that in some areas continued into the 1980s.

As more cardiologists completed training programs and became competent in diagnostic catheterization procedures, the mandate for surgical units or backup within a catheterization facility was relaxed. Invasive cardiologists began to practice in outlying areas, where there was little competition. Eventually, however, they found themselves in markets that lacked the convenience of catheterization facilities, and therefore they began to encourage facilities development.

Invasive cardiologists also enhanced the local noninvasive cardiology capabilities through their ability to interpret results and their insistence on upgraded technology. For example, as echocardiography developed into the preferred diagnostic tool, it grew significantly only in those locations that had a trained cardiologist because the technology needed to interpret results required a cardiologist's specialized skills.

Once departments of cardiology began to develop in these locations, for reasons of economy many were combined with departments of respiratory care. The training is comparable, and the demand for services has supported this arrangement.

In a hospital's medical staff organization, cardiovascular surgeons routinely make up a section within the department of surgery, whereas cardiologists work within the department of medicine. Cardiac anesthesia may function as a section within the anesthesia department.

Some hospitals with large cardiovascular programs have considered the appropriateness of forming an independent department of cardiovascular services. Although there is some efficiency and logic to independent organization, the general response of the organized medical staff is to avoid such centralization because it could result in a concentration of power that might negate the checks and balances currently built into the system. Nonetheless, the future may see an evolution in the direction of increased centralization of CV services.

In most settings, the day-to-day functions of cardiovascular surgery are overseen by the general operating room staff in the surgery department. Although there is often dedicated staff within the operating room, the supervision and management of supplies, for example, are handled by the same management team that directs general surgery. Separate management for cardiac surgery is most often appropriate only for extremely large patient volumes or when the physical facility for cardiac surgery is distinct or allows significant separation.

Cardiac surgery patients typically recover in a dedicated cardiac surgery intensive care unit (CSICU), which essentially is a specialized, postsurgical intensive care unit designed and staffed to facilitate patient recovery and to provide initial postoperative care. Currently, CSICU care lasts from 24 to 72 hours. Here the postoperative patient occupies a bed equipped with telemetry monitoring, which means the nurses can continuously monitor the patient's EKG from their stations. As the patient progresses to a more stable condition, he or she is discharged or transferred to a cardiac/telemetry nursing unit.

Lengths of stay vary widely depending on the program and the type of surgery. Increasingly, patients undergoing cardiac catheterization only are increasingly scheduled on either an outpatient or a 23-hour admission basis. Patients undergoing angioplasty typically spend only one day in the CSICU and a day or two in a monitored bed prior to discharge.

The coronary care unit (CCU), dedicated to nonsurgical patients with cardiovascular diseases, generally is recommended for patients with myocardial infarctions or other suspected cardiac problems. The CCU is staffed by nurses whose training includes recognition of arrhythmia (irregular cardiac rhythm) and treatment of major cardiac problems. A patient is generally transferred to a telemetry unit once he or she has been fully diagnosed or his or her condition has stabilized. The CCU is also dedicated to patients who have already been diagnosed as having serious cardiac disease but for whom no specific procedure has been planned.

Nursing personnel assigned to cardiovascular units typically report through the same structure as all other nursing personnel.

As a rule, medical directors are assigned and often paid for services they perform in the following areas: cardiology, cardiac catheterization, noninvasive cardiology, CSICU, CCU, cardiac rehabilitation, cardiovascular surgery, cardiac anesthesiology, and cardiopulmonology. Their duties vary widely, and compensation is dictated by the competitive environment for cardiologists, the operational environment, and the amount of work required in an area or necessitated by circumstances of the department.

Product Line Management and Cardiovascular Services

Recently, hospitals have made attempts to apply the industrial principle of product or service line management to cardiovascular surgery and services;

the results have been mixed. *Product or service line management* is an organizational strategy that involves restructuring those departments, functions, or services that are related to a particular clinical specialty or subspecialty.

Traditionally, hospitals have been organized in a functional hierarchy in which like services are arranged in departments responsible to department managers and like departments are combined into divisions responsible to vice-presidents. Examples include broad areas such as surgery and pediatrics. In essence product line management (PLM) turns the organization on its side and groups employees not by function but by the *clinical specialty* being provided.

In the case of cardiovascular services, nurses in the operating room, for example, historically have reported to the operating room manager, who in turn reported either to the vice-president for nursing or the vice-president for professional services. However, in a product line management structure, the nurses in the operating room report to a supervisor for cardiovascular surgical services, who in turn reports to a product line manager, who usually functions at the level of vice-president. The cardiovascular services product line manager may also be responsible for the nurses in the CSICU; the CCU; perhaps the telemetry unit; the department of cardiology, including non-invasive cardiology and the cardiac catheterization laboratory; cardiac rehabilitation; and so on. Two principal determinants dictate the success of product or service line management: the skill of the product line manager and the support and organization of the medical staff and the medical directors.

Although the principle of full-fledged product line management sounds reasonable, it is impractical in most settings, given the relative size of many programs and the other responsibilities of those involved. One of several modifications of the concept can make it more practical for daily application. One modification involves developing a program from a group of services.

A *program* is an integrated set of services. Unlike PLM or a matrix organization (discussed in chapter 5), a program is physician-driven. Physician leadership is characterized by a variety of methods — from an autocratic style in which the organization is driven by the will and vision of a single physician, to the alliance of a cardiologist and a cardiovascular surgeon, to the emergence of a single group that fuels the program as a whole, not just individual group practices.

There are, of course, variations on these themes. However, a principal theme of this book is that whereas cardiovascular services or any other clinical service can be run successfully under the inspirational direction and leadership of management, the strongest cardiology programs across the country are most often built around strong physicians. If physicians provide the appropriate level and type of leadership, a program emerges. Program development will be addressed in this context throughout the book.

Summary

Cardiovascular disease is the leading cause of death in the United States. The effort to diagnose and treat it is of great interest to hospitals because of the number of potential patients, the revenue dollars associated with cardiovascular services, the focus cardiovascular disease receives among managed care companies and payers, and the prestige that is currently associated with the provision of CV services.

The principal categories of heart disease are congenital (malfunctions due to birth defects), electrophysiological (conduction impulse irregularities that cause the heartbeat to malfunction), valvular (malfunctions of the valves between the heart chambers), and arterial (plaque buildup in the arteries supplying blood to the heart, which causes the muscle tissue to die).

Cardiologists are internal medicine specialists who diagnose heart disease and, in selected cases, perform procedures to correct certain conditions. Because they intervene in the pathological process, cardiologists who perform these procedures are considered interventional cardiologists. Cardiologists who perform diagnostic cardiac catheterizations are referred to as invasive cardiologists; those who do not are regarded as noninvasive cardiologists.

Historically, cardiovascular services have been organized according to an administrative model. As competition increases and pressures mount, a physician-centered organizational model will be pursued by many hospitals in an effort to build a program.

☐ References

1. American Heart Association. *1991 Heart and Stroke Facts.* Dallas, TX: American Heart Association, 1991.

2. National Center for Health Statistics. *Health, United States, 1989.* Hyattsville, MD: Public Health Service, 1990.

3. National Center for Health Statistics.

4. American Heart Association.

Chapter 2

Dimensions of Change in the Cardiovascular Market

Management is about change and adjusting to change. The role of a manager is to assess external environmental forces and how they bring about change within an organization and then to ensure appropriate response to those forces in an orderly and timely fashion.

Because of rapid changes in cardiovascular services, managers and administrators in health care are faced with the challenge of managing efficiently and cost-effectively in a dynamic environment. This chapter will identify some of the changes in CV services, along with expected trends, and recommend suitable responses to many of them. Discussion will focus on six areas:

- Service trends
- Service projections
- Market maturity
- Strategic program elements
- Physicians as distributors
- Standard treatment protocols

Service Trends

Certain key trends are apparent in CV services:

- Changes in service availability and growth
- Changes in service delivery
- Regulation and payer trends
- Growth of managed care
- Technological advancement

Availability and Growth

The increase in the number of physicians specializing in cardiac medicine has had a significant impact on growth in the field. Two major forces are driving the growing number of hospitals that offer CV services: the influx of cardiologists and their location in communities (such as suburban, semi-rural, and rural markets) previously not served directly by a resident invasive cardiologist. Consequently, these cardiologists have sponsored the addition of cardiovascular technologies in their hospitals, thus paving the way for CV surgery to be performed in locations and at volumes deemed impossible or inappropriate during the 1970s.

The following analysis of the national market for cardiovascular services examines a number of issues, including trends and assumptions within the health care industry, that can be expected to affect future cardiovascular services.

The number of hospitals with cardiovascular surgery programs grew by nearly 32 percent between 1987 and 1990, and the number of hospitals offering cardiac catheterization services increased by nearly 34 percent during this same period (table 2-1). The late 1980s also saw development of mobile cardiac catheterization units and significant growth in the number of freestanding (non–hospital-based) cardiac catheterization laboratories, both of which are projected to increase dramatically during the next decade.

As table 2-1 also demonstrates, the growth of CV programs during the 1980s was significant and widespread. That is, although most states experienced growth in services between 1982 and 1990, the program distribution was notably uneven. Table 2-2 analyzes the state-by-state experiences and then groups the data by geographical regions.

As the population ages, the use rates for all procedures—including cardiovascular surgery—can be expected to increase. However, as payers apply

Table 2-1. U.S. Hospitals Providing Cardiac Catheterization and Cardiovascular Surgery

State	Catheterization			Surgery		
	1982	1987	1990	1982	1987	1990
Alabama	16	24	27	6	14	18
Alaska	4	2	2	2	1	1
Arizona	10	15	21	7	11	20
Arkansas	15	21	23	4	10	12
California	110	139	142	79	98	107
Colorado	15	19	20	12	15	18
Connecticut	15	18	18	6	6	7
Delaware	1	1	2	0	1	1
District of Columbia	8	7	9	6	6	7
Florida	43	46	88	36	39	51

Table 2-1. (Continued)

State	Catheterization			Surgery		
	1982	1987	1990	1982	1987	1990
Georgia	26	31	34	12	12	17
Hawaii	5	5	5	3	2	4
Idaho	3	3	3	1	1	2
Illinois	52	58	77	29	28	42
Indiana	19	24	39	13	14	22
Iowa	12	13	20	7	7	11
Kansas	10	9	13	7	7	11
Kentucky	10	15	27	5	9	12
Louisiana	20	27	39	12	18	30
Maine	4	4	5	1	1	2
Maryland	12	21	30	6	6	7
Massachusetts	20	21	20	11	12	13
Michigan	36	34	50	19	20	26
Minnesota	16	15	16	12	10	16
Mississippi	8	8	13	5	5	9
Missouri	27	36	46	14	21	31
Montana	4	6	8	2	3	4
Nebraska	9	8	13	7	5	8
Nevada	6	5	6	5	3	5
New Hampshire	2	3	9	1	2	2
New Jersey	25	21	25	12	10	13
New Mexico	4	5	5	3	4	4
New York	50	58	56	24	32	27
North Carolina	22	13	36	8	11	17
North Dakota	4	7	7	4	4	6
Ohio	50	53	74	28	30	37
Oklahoma	13	16	19	11	11	14
Oregon	10	15	19	8	9	10
Pennsylvania	46	44	49	33	32	37
Rhode Island	3	2	3	2	2	2
South Carolina	7	11	19	7	8	8
South Dakota	1	1	3	1	1	3
Tennessee	19	21	36	16	12	25
Texas	69	75	113	53	65	89
Utah	8	10	12	6	7	8
Vermont	2	2	1	1	1	1
Virginia	11	15	37	8	6	15
Washington	18	23	29	10	10	12
West Virginia	5	6	13	3	3	4
Wisconsin	22	19	30	17	14	18
Wyoming	3	3	2	2	1	2
Total	930	1,058	1,413	587	660	868
Percentage Increase 1987–1990			33.6%			31.5%
Percentage Increase 1982–1990			51.9%			47.9%

Source: Based on statistics from the *American Hospital Association Guide to the Health Care Field,* 1983, 1988, 1991 editions.

Table 2-2.   U.S. Hospitals Providing Cardiac Catheterization and Cardiovascular Surgery by Region

Region	Catheterization			Surgery		
	1982	1987	1990	1982	1987	1990
Far West:						
Washington	18	23	29	10	10	12
Oregon	10	15	19	8	9	10
California	110	139	142	79	98	107
Nevada	6	5	6	5	3	5
Idaho	3	3	3	1	1	2
Montana	4	6	8	2	3	4
Wyoming	3	3	2	2	1	2
Utah	8	10	12	6	7	8
Arizona	10	15	21	7	11	20
New Mexico	4	5	5	3	4	4
Colorado	15	19	20	12	15	18
Alaska	4	2	2	2	1	1
Hawaii	5	5	5	3	2	4
Total	200	250	274	140	165	197
Near West:						
North Dakota	4	7	7	4	4	6
South Dakota	1	1	3	1	1	3
Nebraska	9	8	13	7	5	8
Kansas	10	9	13	7	7	11
Oklahoma	13	16	19	11	11	14
Texas	69	75	113	53	65	89
Louisiana	20	27	39	12	18	30
Arkansas	15	21	23	4	10	12
Missouri	27	36	46	14	21	31
Iowa	12	13	20	7	7	11
Minnesota	16	15	16	12	10	16
Total	196	228	312	132	159	231
South:						
Mississippi	8	8	13	5	5	9
Alabama	16	24	27	6	14	18
Georgia	26	31	34	12	12	17
Florida	43	46	88	36	39	51
North Carolina	22	13	36	8	11	17
South Carolina	7	11	19	7	8	8
Virginia	11	15	37	8	6	15
Tennessee	19	21	36	16	12	25
Kentucky	10	15	27	5	9	12
West Virginia	5	6	13	3	3	4
Maryland	12	21	30	6	6	7
Delaware	1	1	2	0	1	1
District of Columbia	8	7	9	6	6	7
Total	188	219	371	118	132	191

Table 2-2. (Continued)

Region	Catheterization			Surgery		
	1982	1987	1990	1982	1987	1990
East North Central:						
Wisconsin	22	19	30	17	14	18
Michigan	36	34	50	19	20	26
Illinois	52	58	77	29	28	42
Indiana	19	24	39	13	14	22
Ohio	50	53	74	28	30	37
Total	179	188	270	106	106	145
Northeast:						
New York	50	58	56	24	32	27
Pennsylvania	46	44	49	33	32	37
New Jersey	25	21	25	12	10	13
Connecticut	15	18	18	6	6	7
Massachusetts	20	21	20	11	12	13
Vermont	2	2	1	1	1	1
New Hampshire	2	3	9	1	2	2
Maine	4	4	5	1	1	2
Rhode Island	3	2	3	2	2	2
Total	167	173	186	91	98	104
Summary:						
Far West	200	250	274	140	165	197
Near West	196	228	312	132	159	231
South	188	219	371	118	132	191
East North Central	179	188	270	106	106	145
Northeast	167	173	186	91	98	104
Total	930	1,058	1,413	587	660	868

Source: Based on statistics from the *American Hospital Association Guide to the Health Care Field,* 1983, 1988, 1991 editions.

stronger measures to reduce the cost of health care and as less-invasive procedures become increasingly effective, the incidence rates for surgery can be projected to decrease. These countervailing trends should result in stable use rates for cardiovascular surgery and other cardiac procedures.

By dividing population figures by the total number of cardiovascular programs, one can calculate roughly the population served by each hospital that has a cardiac catheterization laboratory and cardiac surgery program. This information is displayed by state in table 2-3 and by region in table 2-4. Tables 2-5 and 2-6 rank the states by the size of population served for hospitals with catheterization laboratories and surgery programs, respectively.

In 1990 the average population served by a hospital with a cardiac catheterization program (which may include more than one catheterization laboratory and excludes freestanding and mobile catheterization laboratories) was

Table 2-3. Distribution of Cardiovascular Programs by State: 1990

State	Total State Population	Hospitals with Catheterization Laboratories	Population Served by Hospital	Cardiovascular Surgery Programs	Population Served by Hospital
Alabama	4,062,608	27	150,467	18	225,700
Alaska	551,947	2	275,974	1	551,947
Arizona	3,677,985	21	175,142	20	183,899
Arkansas	2,362,239	23	102,706	12	196,853
California	29,839,250	142	210,136	107	278,871
Colorado	3,307,912	20	165,396	18	183,773
Connecticut	3,295,669	18	183,093	7	470,810
Delaware	668,696	2	334,348	1	668,696
District of Columbia	621,850	9	69,094	7	88,836
Florida	13,003,362	88	147,765	51	254,968
Georgia	6,508,419	34	191,424	17	382,848
Hawaii	1,115,274	5	223,055	4	278,819
Idaho	1,011,986	3	347,329	2	520,993
Illinois	11,466,682	77	148,918	42	273,016
Indiana	5,564,228	39	142,673	22	252,919
Iowa	2,787,424	20	139,371	11	253,402
Kansas	2,485,600	13	191,200	11	225,964
Kentucky	3,698,969	27	136,999	12	308,247
Louisiana	4,238,216	39	108,672	30	141,274
Maine	1,233,223	5	246,645	2	616,612
Maryland	4,798,622	30	159,954	7	685,517
Massachusetts	6,029,051	20	301,453	13	463,773
Michigan	9,328,784	50	186,576	26	358,799
Minnesota	4,387,029	16	274,189	16	274,189
Mississippi	2,586,443	13	198,957	9	287,383
Missouri	5,137,804	46	111,691	31	165,736
Montana	803,665	8	100,458	4	200,916
Nebraska	1,584,617	13	121,894	8	198,077
Nevada	1,206,152	6	201,025	5	241,230
New Hampshire	1,113,915	9	123,768	2	556,958
New Jersey	7,748,634	25	309,945	13	596,049
New Mexico	1,521,779	5	304,356	4	380,445
New York	18,044,505	56	322,223	27	668,315
North Carolina	6,657,630	36	184,934	17	391,625
North Dakota	641,364	7	91,623	6	106,894
Ohio	10,887,325	74	147,126	37	294,252
Oklahoma	3,157,604	19	166,190	14	225,543
Oregon	2,853,733	19	150,196	10	285,373
Pennsylvania	11,924,710	49	243,361	37	322,289
Rhode Island	1,005,984	3	335,328	2	502,992
South Carolina	3,505,707	19	184,511	8	438,213
South Dakota	699,999	3	233,333	3	233,333
Tennessee	4,896,641	36	136,018	25	195,866
Texas	17,059,805	113	150,972	89	191,683
Utah	1,727,784	12	143,982	8	215,973
Vermont	564,964	1	564,964	1	564,964
Virginia	6,216,568	37	168,015	15	414,438
Washington	4,887,941	29	168,550	12	407,328
West Virginia	1,801,625	13	138,587	4	450,406
Wisconsin	4,906,745	30	163,558	18	272,597
Wyoming	455,975	2	227,988	2	227,988
Total	249,644,643	1,413	176,679	868	287,612

Sources: Based on statistics from the *American Hospital Association Guide to the Health Care Field*, 1991 edition; and U.S. Census Bureau.

Table 2-4. Distribution of Selected Cardiovascular Programs by Region: 1990

Region	Regional Population	Hospitals with Catheterization Laboratories	Population Served by Hospital	Cardiovascular Surgery Programs	Population Served by Hospital
Far West	52,961,383	274	193,290	197	268,840
Near West	44,541,701	312	142,762	231	192,821
South	59,027,140	371	159,103	191	309,043
East North Central	42,153,764	270	156,125	145	290,716
Northeast	50,960,655	186	273,982	104	490,006

Sources: Based on statistics from the *American Hospital Association Guide to the Health Care Field,* 1991 edition; and U.S. Census Bureau.

176,679 (table 2-5), and the average population served per cardiovascular surgery program was 287,612 (table 2-6). These figures are equivalent to estimated average hospital per-program (*not* per–catheterization-laboratory) volumes of 763 catheterizations and 443 cardiovascular surgeries, based on the gross national figures for the most recent year for which such figures were available (see tables 1-6 and 1-8 for national utilization rates).

Although these calculations yield only gross figures, they do underscore the wide differences in populations served. For example, table 2-6 demonstrates that despite Texas and New York having similar populations, Texas has more than three times the number of cardiac surgery programs (89 versus New York's 27). California has the largest number of surgery programs (107), but nearly 60 percent of California's programs are in the Greater Los Angeles area. As a result, there are more cardiac surgery programs in the three-county Los Angeles area than in the entire state of New York, and Texas is the only state with more surgical programs than the Los Angeles area.

These overall growth patterns are important because, according to some authorities, they improve the access, availability, and competitiveness of cardiovascular services. Yet these same patterns are bemoaned by others as both indicating and contributing to the commercialization of cardiovascular services, presenting a recipe for disaster by decreasing average program case volume and, presumably, clinical quality. As the number of programs increases faster than case volume, the average per-program activity decreases.

It is not the purpose of this book to debate the appropriate distribution of cardiovascular services. Strong cases can be made by clinicians and policymakers on both sides of the issue. It is important, however, to recognize that virtually all medical technologies and procedures advance through a product life cycle that results in their becoming more widely available. For example, this is the case with transplantation procedures, which have become more widely used. Therefore, it is predictable that CV services will continue to follow this trend of technology dissemination and become increasingly

Table 2-5.   State Ranking by Population per Catheterization
Laboratory: 1990

State	State Population	Hospitals with Catheterization Laboratories	Population Served by Hospital
District of Columbia	621,850	9	69,094
North Dakota	641,364	7	91,623
Montana	803,665	8	100,458
Arkansas	2,362,239	23	102,706
Louisiana	4,238,216	39	108,672
Missouri	5,137,804	46	111,691
Nebraska	1,584,617	13	121,894
New Hampshire	1,113,915	9	123,768
Tennessee	4,896,641	36	136,018
Kentucky	3,698,969	27	136,999
West Virginia	1,801,625	13	138,587
Iowa	2,787,424	20	139,371
Indiana	5,564,228	39	142,673
Utah	1,727,784	12	143,982
Ohio	10,887,325	74	147,126
Florida	13,003,362	88	147,765
Illinois	11,466,682	77	148,918
Oregon	2,853,733	19	150,196
Alabama	4,062,608	27	150,467
Texas	17,059,805	113	150,972
Maryland	4,798,622	30	159,954
Wisconsin	4,906,745	30	163,558
Colorado	3,307,912	20	165,396
Oklahoma	3,157,604	19	166,190
Virginia	6,216,568	37	168,015
Washington	4,887,941	29	168,550
Arizona	3,677,985	21	175,142
Connecticut	3,295,669	18	183,093
South Carolina	3,505,707	19	184,511
North Carolina	6,657,630	36	184,934
Michigan	9,328,784	50	186,576
Kansas	2,485,600	13	191,200
Georgia	6,508,419	34	191,424
Mississippi	2,586,443	13	198,957
Nevada	1,206,152	6	201,025
California	29,839,250	142	210,136
Hawaii	1,115,274	5	223,055
Wyoming	455,975	2	227,988
South Dakota	699,999	3	233,333
Pennsylvania	11,924,710	49	243,361
Maine	1,233,223	5	246,645
Minnesota	4,387,029	16	274,189
Alaska	551,947	2	275,974
Massachusetts	6,029,051	20	301,453
New Mexico	1,521,779	5	304,356
New Jersey	7,748,634	25	309,945
New York	18,044,505	56	322,223
Delaware	668,696	2	334,348
Rhode Island	1,005,984	3	335,328
Idaho	1,011,986	3	347,329
Vermont	564,964	1	564,964
Total	249,644,643	1,413	176,679

Sources: Based on statistics from the *American Hospital Association Guide to the Health Care Field*, 1991 edition; and U.S. Census Bureau.

Table 2-6. State Ranking by Population per Cardiovascular Surgery Program: 1990

State	State Population	Hospitals with Cardiovascular Surgery Programs	Population Served by Hospital
District of Columbia	621,850	7	88,836
North Dakota	641,364	6	106,894
Louisiana	4,238,216	30	141,274
Missouri	5,137,804	31	165,736
Colorado	3,307,912	18	183,773
Arizona	3,677,985	20	183,899
Texas	17,059,805	89	191,683
Tennessee	4,896,641	25	195,866
Arkansas	2,362,239	12	196,853
Nebraska	1,584,617	8	198,077
Montana	803,665	4	200,916
Utah	1,727,784	8	215,973
Oklahoma	3,157,604	14	225,543
Alabama	4,062,608	18	225,700
Kansas	2,485,600	11	225,964
Wyoming	455,975	2	227,988
South Dakota	699,999	3	233,333
Nevada	1,206,152	5	241,230
Indiana	5,564,228	22	252,919
Iowa	2,787,424	11	253,402
Florida	13,003,362	51	254,968
Wisconsin	4,906,745	18	272,597
Illinois	11,466,682	42	273,016
Minnesota	4,387,029	16	274,189
Hawaii	1,115,274	4	278,819
California	29,839,750	107	278,871
Oregon	2,853,733	10	285,373
Mississippi	2,586,443	9	287,383
Ohio	10,887,325	37	294,252
Kentucky	3,698,969	12	308,247
Pennsylvania	11,924,710	37	322,289
Michigan	9,328,784	26	358,799
New Mexico	1,521,779	4	380,445
Georgia	6,508,419	17	382,848
North Carolina	6,657,630	17	391,625
Washington	4,887,941	12	407,328
Virginia	6,216,568	15	414,438
South Carolina	3,505,707	8	438,213
West Virginia	1,801,625	4	450,406
Massachusetts	6,029,051	13	463,773
Connecticut	3,295,669	7	470,810
Rhode Island	1,005,984	2	502,992
Idaho	1,011,986	2	520,993
Alaska	551,947	1	551,947
New Hampshire	1,113,915	2	556,958
Vermont	564,964	1	564,964
New Jersey	7,748,634	13	596,049
Maine	1,233,223	2	616,612
Maryland	4,798,622	7	685,517
New York	18,044,505	27	668,315
Delaware	668,696	1	668,696
Total	249,644,643	868	287,612

Sources: Based on statistics from the *American Hospital Association Guide to the Health Care Field*, 1991 edition; and U.S. Census Bureau.

available at more, and smaller, institutions. Hospitals enjoying large volumes today must anticipate increased competition from new entrants to the market, and hospitals without cardiovascular surgery and invasive cardiology programs must continue to evaluate the appropriateness of these services for their institutions and their communities.

Although similarities exist among most cardiovascular markets, it is beneficial to examine the macro trends in the industry, compare those trends with the realities of the local market, and plan appropriate responses to the changes in both the internal and the external environments. A program assessment model is shown in chapter 3 (figure 3-1), along with guidelines for assessing the internal and local environments.

Medical care is subject to many market influences and trends. This may be even more true in cardiovascular services because they represent both the major revenue source for providers and the most costly disease entity for payers (estimated to represent as much as 30 percent of their expenditures). This results in cardiac care being a major focus of both provider and payer attention, innovative policy modification, and resource allocation. On the basis of the number of dollars in the cardiovascular market, there is considerable interest in managing the flow of patients and funds within the market. This suggests a future with the probability of significant upheaval.

Delivery of Service

The principal concern for the future of cardiovascular service delivery is the potential for regionalization, especially for cardiovascular surgery. This concern became acute with the genesis of the Health Care Financing Administration (HCFA) concept of centers of excellence and the potential for improving quality while saving money. The centers of excellence concept arose as a logical result of hospitals' having attained distinctive competencies in certain specialized services. Although the clustering of talent and development of competencies is a natural phenomenon, not until the early 1980s did the phrase first emerge in the Southwest and become popularized in the mid-1980s by a national health insurer. The concept quickly became a marketing and program development catchphrase. Soon every hospital had one or more centers of excellence (or, more appropriately, centers of attention).

The HCFA's interest in centers of excellence has increased interest in the concept. The agency's Demonstration Project in Cardiovascular Surgery, which in 1991 designated six hospitals nationally as participants, is expected by many to set the trend for further centralization in the 1990s, not only for CV services but for other high-cost specialty services as well.

Other programs, such as specialty preferred provider organizations (SPPOs) and carve-out HMOs, are also expected to hasten the trend toward centralization of services. These entities will develop networks of exclusive specialty providers in large geographic areas. The patients of participating employers and payers will be channeled through these networks.

The centralization of specialty services has a certain intellectual soundness to it. Whereas centralization will help strong programs to get stronger — particularly when they are located in an attractive market — it is unlikely that this trend will return the delivery system to anything that resembles what was in place during the 1970s. This is principally because the strong programs of the 1970s generally are not located in communities that will be able to support them in the 1990s. The future will include more successful programs in new geographic locations in large metropolitan markets, as smaller suburban providers expand and inner-city providers broaden their markets through satellite facilities and business relationships with suburban providers.

The centralization of cardiovascular services is in direct opposition to the natural trend for technology to disseminate and become more widely available in response to providers' and patients' interest in having services more conveniently located. Central to the needs of both communities is convenience in the purchase of medical services.

Much of the current emphasis on the centralization of care in cardiovascular services is based on wide differences in *cost* of care. In California, for example, the average patient charge for open-heart surgery at established centers for a bypass procedure (DRG [diagnosis-related group] 107) ranged from less than $6,000 to more than $90,000 in 1988. See table 2-7. These variations are not explained by program size or quality. Some of the largest and most prestigious programs in California are among the most costly, and several low-volume programs report the lowest average case price. Some of the variation may be explained by case severity or complexity, but this is not the principal determinant. Those programs that have achieved significant price advantage have done so by combining a highly competent team of physicians focused on case price and organized to modify physician behavior around this issue.

Price differences of this magnitude likely will not last. The centers of excellence approach suggests that the inefficient providers will be "regulated out." It can be expected that costs will be brought down to a point of reasonable variation in most markets through cost-reduction techniques such as standard treatment protocols.

Differences in *quality* of care are more difficult to characterize. Quality increasingly will become a focus of attention, and programs will be needed that *manage quality and document results.* These efforts will include closer scrutiny of difficult cases and expanded efforts to work with only highly skilled cardiac physicians.

As hospitals compete more on the basis of quality and cost, they will recognize even further the importance of their medical staff. Also, more aggressive methods for screening less-competent physicians from the medical staff, restricting their privileges, or excluding them from certain contracting initiatives will be developed.

Table 2-7. Comparison of Case Prices and Volume for Bypass Procedure (DRG 107): California, 1988

Ranked by Price per Case			Ranked by Volume of Cases		
Number of Cases	Average Length of Stay	Average Case Price	Number of Cases	Average Length of Stay	Average Case Price
16	15.4	$91,039	541	10.4	$35,443
39	15.4	$76,873	386	12.0	$38,303
26	14.0	$74,015	385	10.5	$40,691
20	11.6	$62,395	384	12.8	$39,855
177	13.6	$59,839	365	10.2	$39,433
21	11.0	$59,805	263	9.2	$34,391
37	13.8	$59,496	241	11.6	$58,054
241	11.6	$58,054	236	9.7	$26,323
17	10.9	$51,768	223	10.9	$29,725
16	9.8	$49,363	216	9.8	$31,351
114	12.6	$49,170	213	13.6	$48,404
21	12.7	$48,646	196	9.9	$31,998
72	13.8	$48,465	184	10.1	$29,501
213	13.6	$48,404	177	13.6	$59,839
90	10.4	$47,930	176	11.1	$43,461
13	7.5	$46,467	163	10.3	$45,583
6	13.3	$46,069	156	9.1	$25,005
36	11.3	$45,785	141	9.5	$30,092
163	10.3	$45,583	132	10.7	$37,701
23	14.5	$44,827	127	9.4	$32,086
75	9.4	$44,715	126	9.5	$29,324
89	10.4	$44,079	126	9.6	$35,807
21	11.1	$44,074	114	12.6	$49,170
68	12.0	$43,935	108	11.1	$36,234
38	10.5	$43,669	102	11.2	$33,150
82	15.2	$43,662	101	10.5	$42,991
176	11.1	$43,461	98	10.2	$35,754
101	10.5	$42,991	96	11.7	$32,947
48	11.3	$42,880	95	12.6	$31,188
12	8.8	$42,645	94	13.7	$30,125
31	9.7	$42,388	90	10.4	$47,930
76	11.7	$41,881	89	10.4	$44,079
46	10.3	$41,265	85	11.0	$29,734
63	9.1	$40,813	85	9.8	$32,171
33	9.3	$40,775	84	8.7	$26,466
385	10.5	$40,691	83	11.4	$32,499
63	11.0	$40,569	83	9.5	$29,032
33	11.2	$40,324	82	15.2	$43,662
33	9.6	$40,245	82	8.2	$25,950
5	8.0	$39,960	78	9.7	$34,266
38	10.8	$39,882	76	11.7	$41,881
384	12.8	$39,855	75	9.4	$44,715
365	10.2	$39,433	75	8.4	$24,822
47	10.6	$39,221	73	10.7	$33,282
28	9.6	$39,001	72	13.8	$48,465

Table 2-7. (Continued)

Ranked by Price per Case			Ranked by Volume of Cases		
Number of Cases	Average Length of Stay	Average Case Price	Number of Cases	Average Length of Stay	Average Case Price
51	12.0	$38,853	70	8.5	$34,885
386	12.0	$38,303	68	12.0	$43,935
34	12.2	$38,076	65	9.2	$24,368
132	10.7	$37,701	63	9.5	$34,777
42	9.8	$37,624	63	9.1	$40,813
52	9.4	$37,426	63	11.0	$40,569
15	10.4	$36,985	56	12.9	$33,746
108	11.1	$36,234	55	11.0	$34,018
126	9.6	$35,807	52	10.7	$33,363
43	11.1	$35,763	52	9.8	$32,072
98	10.2	$35,754	52	8.8	$32,585
541	10.4	$35,443	52	9.4	$37,426
70	8.5	$34,885	51	19.9	$31,458
13	9.3	$34,819	51	12.0	$38,853
63	9.5	$34,777	51	10.2	$31,471
43	11.4	$34,717	49	10.5	$31,109
18	10.3	$34,689	49	10.3	$31,938
263	9.2	$34,391	48	11.3	$42,880
78	9.7	$34,266	48	17.2	$23,179
16	10.5	$34,247	47	10.6	$39,221
55	11.0	$34,018	47	8.6	$29,930
56	12.9	$33,746	46	10.3	$41,265
5	8.4	$33,731	43	11.4	$34,717
52	10.7	$33,363	43	11.1	$35,763
73	10.7	$33,282	42	9.8	$37,624
102	11.2	$33,150	39	15.4	$76,873
96	11.7	$32,947	38	10.5	$43,669
52	8.8	$32,585	38	10.8	$39,882
83	11.4	$32,499	37	13.8	$59,496
85	9.8	$32,171	36	11.3	$45,785
127	9.4	$32,086	34	12.2	$38,076
52	9.8	$32,072	33	9.6	$40,245
196	9.9	$31,998	33	9.3	$40,775
49	10.3	$31,938	33	11.2	$40,324
51	10.2	$31,471	31	9.7	$42,388
51	19.9	$31,458	28	9.6	$39,001
216	9.8	$31,351	26	14.0	$74,015
95	12.6	$31,188	23	14.5	$44,827
49	10.5	$31,109	22	10.9	$27,572
94	13.7	$30,125	21	11.0	$59,805
141	9.5	$30,092	21	11.1	$44,074
47	8.6	$29,930	21	12.7	$48,646
85	11.0	$29,734	20	11.6	$62,395
223	10.9	$29,725	18	10.3	$34,689

(Continued on next page)

Table 2-7.   (Continued)

Ranked by Price per Case			Ranked by Volume of Cases		
Number of Cases	Average Length of Stay	Average Case Price	Number of Cases	Average Length of Stay	Average Case Price
184	10.1	$29,501	17	10.9	$51,768
126	9.5	$29,324	16	10.5	$34,247
83	9.5	$29,032	16	9.8	$49,363
22	10.9	$27,572	16	15.4	$91,039
84	8.7	$26,466	16	10.3	$25,283
236	9.7	$26,323	16	10.3	$25,283
82	8.2	$25,950	15	10.4	$36,985
16	10.3	$25,283	13	9.3	$34,819
16	10.3	$25,283	13	7.5	$46,467
156	9.1	$25,005	12	8.8	$42,645
75	8.4	$24,822	6	13.3	$46,069
65	9.2	$24,368	5	8.0	$39,960
48	17.2	$23,179	5	8.4	$33,731
1	7.0	$22,351	1	4.0	$5,155
1	9.0	$18,749	1	7.0	$22,351
1	4.0	$5,155	1	9.0	$18,749

Source: California Office of Statewide Health Planning and Development.

Small and developing programs will face an increased challenge to compete on the basis of quality and cost. Already it is evident that a relatively small program can be both price and quality competitive — provided that the appropriate physicians are involved with the program.

The ability of small programs to compete in cardiovascular services is a recent phenomenon. As CV services mature and become more commonplace, the qualitative differences between the high-volume, urban program and the community hospital program with smaller volumes will be less apparent.

Once quality and cost are comparable, *consumer convenience* is the next-most-important determining factor in service delivery. Just as with consumer products, convenience or location plays a surprisingly important role. It is predictable that, despite an initial struggle between the large established programs and developing ones, program success most likely will rest on location rather than on historical dominance. In most urban markets, this suggests redistributing programs away from the downtown setting and moving large urban hospitals into the suburban and semirural markets.

Regulations and Payers

The proliferation of cardiovascular programs can be seen as either a trend motivated by greed or as a natural evolution of the delivery system. The two sides are at odds most pointedly on the issue of volume-related regulation.

In California this issue was recently considered in a revision of the California administrative code covering cardiovascular programs. The effort to rewrite the statutes regulating cardiovascular services was in part a response to a legislative initiative to close by regulation those programs performing fewer than 150 or 200 cardiac surgeries per year and to prevent new programs from being approved should they fail to demonstrate volumes in excess of that threshold. This legislation was sponsored by several hospitals that had a medium volume of open-heart surgery programs and recognized that they would benefit from the closure of the low-volume programs nearby. Rhetoric focused on the relationship of quality and volume. Those favoring the legislation based their support on the assumption that more (that is, more procedures per year) is always better.

In an interesting administrative breakthrough, the sides compromised, using language that calls for a quality audit to be performed should volume fall below a certain minimum and for action to be taken only should mortality exceed the state average by a given percentage. Further, any program whose mortality fell below this threshold, regardless of its volume, would be subject to audit. This is a posture that regulators can be expected to take in the future; they will be measuring (or at least attempting to measure) the appropriate variable: program quality, not program volume.

When concerns exist over the costs of low-volume programs, a similar approach will be taken. Rather than regulating volume requirements, the price paid for the services will be based on market factors, thereby forcing inefficient providers out of competitive markets.

Two trends of interest in this regard result from joint Medicare and HCFA initiatives. First, Medicare has initiated a pilot program for cardiovascular surgery in which it has entered into contractual arrangements with a handful of centers across the country. As of this writing, these arrangements do not affect referrals to other programs, providing only for discounted, one-price agreements that include the physicians' fees. It is the intent of Medicare to evaluate the effectiveness of regionalizing CV surgery to reduce costs and improve quality. Should this project be deemed effective, it is conceivable that the Medicare conditions of participation could be changed to allow only providers participating in these selective contracts to be reimbursed for cardiovascular surgery. Other high-cost specialized services would then follow this pattern. Although this situation is possible, it is not likely given the history of similar efforts (Comprehensive Health Planning and PL93-641).

A more reasonable approach can be expected that will involve the reduction of case prices or DRG payments based on market conditions and the potential to deny payment to programs for which mortality or other evolving quality measurements do not meet Medicare standards.

A question remains as to which alternative ultimately will reduce the cost of cardiac surgery to the consumer. The increased availability of cardio-vascular services would suggest that service prices (both hospital and physician fees) should be falling. This expanded supply should increase the level of competition, and to the extent that hospitals will compete in the future on the basis of price, the price should fall as a result of this competition. But the economies of scale that presumably result from regionalization and cardiac centers suggest that this would be the less costly alternative.[1]

The complexity of cardiac surgery will be at the center of the debate over regulation versus regionalization. Many physicians contend that quality improves as a result of competition and that cardiac surgery has evolved to the extent that it requires no more regulation than general surgery. If CV surgery is to be considered a common surgical procedure in the sense that it can be performed safely at relatively low volumes in small community hospitals, it will be regulated no more and no less than any other surgical procedure.

The prices of cardiac surgery will reach equilibrium on local, regional, and, to a certain extent, national levels. Competition will ensure this, and smaller programs will be successful in the long term only to the extent that they can approximate the market price. Local program prices will *not* be required to match regional or national prices to be successful because the market determinate of value is a combination of price, quality, and convenience.

Growth of Managed Care

Managed care will be a force in organizing competition for cardiovascular services. Payers and employers faced with insurance rate hikes in excess of 35 percent are pushing for effective methods to control health care costs. The National Association of Manufacturers estimates that the average business spends nearly 37 percent of its net profits on health care costs.[1] As payers look to control costs, they will be looking closely at cardiovascular care because it represents such a large percentage of their total costs.

Conventional managed care has evolved from simple price discounting and per diem pricing to the formation of preferred provider organizations (PPOs) and the combination of hospital fees with physician fees into a single package price. Not only have utilization review and case management spawned new hospital departments, they have created an entirely new industrial segment in health care sales and services to hospitals and payers. Because payers have become more sophisticated in the channeling of patients, the centers of excellence concept has emerged as the most elaborate form of managed care.

The evolution of managed care is continuing in the development of SPPOs or specialty networks. These organizations, focusing initially on cardiac surgery, will create networks of providers in geographically dispersed areas based on the enrolled population of participating payers and employers. In exchange for a committed volume of patients, payers will require low prices. These SPPOs will be successful in channeling patients where traditional PPOs have not been because payers are willing to impose increasingly severe benefit sanctions, including benefit mandates or no coverage for care received by a beneficiary out of the network. These are severe measures that payers are now willing to consider and that many unions even support.

There is an opportunity for hospitals to respond quickly to this new demand by payers. This opportunity has much greater potential than in the past because, although the criteria for contracting will continue to be based on highly competitive standards, the resulting relationship will be collaborative and beneficial to both parties in a way it never was in the past.

Payers are seeking to establish collaborative relationships with hospital and physician providers that will allow them to develop new solutions to old problems. These solutions will be found only when both sides participate as a team and examine the issues from one another's perspectives. It is also important to note that payers are increasingly forcing collaboration between hospitals and physicians in the contracting arena. Figure 2-1 illustrates that all of the recent innovations in managed care contracting either prefer or require hospital–physician collaboration.

Payers will be searching for methods to purchase services on the basis of the following criteria:

- The provider's reputation for quality in a specific product line or service
- A high level of patient satisfaction
- The reputation, education, and specifically related experience of individual physicians and hospital personnel in particular product lines

Figure 2-1. Hospital Reimbursement Trends

	Physician Involvement	
	Required	Preferred
Discounts		
Fixed Fee Schedules		
Per Diem		
Per Case		
Capitation		
HMOs	X	
PPOs		X
Total Package Pricing	X	
Direct Employer Contracting		X
SPPOs	X	

- The program's mortality rate
- The program's infection rate and other indicators of preventable complications
- The volume of procedures in the product line during the past 12 months
- The provider's ability to measure and document quality
- The provider's commitment to the ongoing monitoring and improvement of quality as it relates to the hospital and medical team
- A competitive (low) documented case rate, including hospital and physician charges, that shows a profit margin for the provider

Although the future promises opportunities for those hospitals able to document high-quality and efficient services, the days of payers contracting with hospitals to provide full services for a geographic area are not completely gone. This historical model can be predicted to continue until the collaborative model replaces it. Unfortunately for those who see this as perpetuating the status quo and who fail to seize the opportunities to specialize, document, and collaborate in providing care, there will be a steady erosion of the more desirable services by competition from other providers. In addition, the conventional model that has proved unprofitable in the past will become even more unprofitable in the next few years.

Not surprisingly, many hospitals have misread this new trend and see the relief from including certain high-cost services (such as open-heart surgery) in their per diem managed care rates as positive. Many are proud to have carved out their tertiary services from their per diem so they can be paid their charges (or discounts from charges) for these services. That is not the payers' intention, however. Many contractors allow hospitals to persuade them *not* to include these services so that the payer can later contract for them separately with a high-quality specialty provider that can offer an extremely competitive rate.

A unique opportunity may now exist for many hospitals to position themselves as key providers for one or more specialty areas, including cardiovascular services. Of course, those hospitals that currently are "hospitals of choice" will have the first opportunities to position their services; otherwise, another hospital could position itself as the primary provider of cardiac services. For example, one leading tertiary hospital persuaded the managed care company to exclude their already-profitable cardiac program from the contract but still list the hospital as a preferred provider. This opened the door for another hospital to position itself as the primary provider of cardiac services for managed care patients. Sometimes, the defined service areas for the specialty tertiary products may be larger than for the full-service contract service areas. Hospitals otherwise viewed as high-quality providers may be excluded from a specialty service market because of a specialty provider.

Top hospital managers can be proactive or reactive in responding to changes in managed care. Some will choose a response on the basis of their corporate environment. Others will choose on the basis of their understanding of the institution's readiness and ability to respond. Still others will choose on the basis of the facility's overall mission and goals. A *strategic response* takes all these variables into account and begins with a clear and pragmatic review of each hospital's current strengths and weaknesses. A hospital may not be ready to take a proactive position externally until it puts the internal position in order—which in itself is a proactive step.

Depending on the hospital's current position in the general contracting arena, some hospitals may enjoy the luxury of being sought out by managed care companies currently promoting the specialty program networks (SPPOs, national specialty networks, centers for excellence, institute of quality, HMO specialty designate, and so forth). Perhaps these hospitals can afford to wait to be approached; others, however, will have to be more proactive. New managed care programs potentially are based on exclusivity and long-term contractual relationships. Hospitals that wait may not have another contracting opportunity for years. However, there is time now for hospitals to decide how to participate in these developing specialty managed care relationships.

New Technology

Along with increased cost competition will come increased technological advancements that reduce the rate of surgical procedures. This trend will include a rise in the number and type of interventional procedures performed in the catheterization laboratory, increased use of noncatheterization diagnostic examinations, and a growth in electrophysiologic procedures.

All technology becomes more accessible as it matures, and medical technology is no exception. For example, copy machines, computers, and facsimile machines quickly became commonplace in office environments. The technology of cardiovascular services has evolved in the same way in the health care environment. Major clinical technologies—computed tomographic (CT) scanning, lithotripsy, magnetic resonance imaging (MRI), and the like—all dispersed quickly throughout the community setting. For example, MRI technology was first made commercially available to community hospitals in 1983, and within five years it was available routinely in virtually every U.S. community—if not in a fixed-base site, then through a mobile service.

In contrast, cardiac catheterization technology has been available since the late 1960s but has dispersed slowly. This initial slow growth has been due in part to the depth of organizational commitment required and the preparation an institution must undertake to offer backup CV services as well as to address the comparative severity of illness of many cardiovascular

patients. Nevertheless, cardiac catheterization did become a popular technology for community hospitals by the 1980s, largely because invasive cardiologists, upon locating in smaller hospitals, created the demand for cardiac
catheterization laboratories and cardiovascular surgery programs. Cardiac
catheterization laboratories will continue to be an important technology for
hospitals as catheterization equipment becomes more and more the focus
of practice and the center of diagnosis and treatment. (See chapter 9 for
a more detailed discussion of the technology used in catheterization laboratories.) Related technologies that will continue to grow are listed below:

- *Electrophysiology,* a therapy that takes place in the catheterization
  laboratory, promises to become much more common in the future.
- *Balloon angioplasty (PTCA)* involves fitting a balloon to the end of
  a catheter and inserting it into a plaque-blocked artery. Once the balloon is inflated, the blocked artery will open, thereby reinstating blood
  supply to the heart muscle. This procedure eliminates the need for
  surgically grafting a vein onto the vessel and bypassing the blockage.
- *Pharmaceutical and biotechnological product development* can be
  expected to continue.
- *Laser catheterization,* which involves eliminating plaque buildup
  through the use of lasers, shows promise but is developing slowly.
- *Atherectomy,* which involves attaching a grinding device to the end
  of a catheter for the removal of plaque buildup, shows more immediate promise than laser catheterization, but PTCA will remain the principal interventional technique used in cardiac catheterization
  laboratories for the foreseeable future.

Alternative diagnostic therapies will become better understood. For example, cardiac ultrasound (echocardiography/cardiac doppler), transesophageal
echocardiography (TEE), ultrafast computed tomography (CT), and positron
emission tomography (PET) all hold promise for advancing cardiac imaging.
For the foreseeable future, PET will continue to be so expensive that only very
large centers will be able to afford the technology. Thus, PET should be monitored for price viability as well as the improvements in the technology that
may represent either a threat of competition or an opportunity.

Interventional cardiology is presently tied to the surgery suite through
standard-of-practice conventions linked to patient safety, but it is predictable that the relationship between interventional cardiology and surgery will
change and eventually be broken. Technologies such as vascular stents (mesh
tubes used to keep arteries open) and left ventricular assist devices (LVADs)
will eventually allow angioplasty to be performed without requiring cardiac
surgery as a backup. Simple angioplasties (generally involving low-risk
patients with single-vessel disease) are performed increasingly with a surgical team available but not standing by.

A gradual and steady loosening of the requirements that tie some procedures to cardiac surgery is currently creating the potential for major market changes. This may be the necessary precursor to a consolidation in the cardiac surgery market. It is conceivable (though unprecedented) that, because the underlying economies will have changed, hospitals could leave the cardiac surgery market over the next five years at a rate that equals or exceeds the rate at which they recently entered the market. At present, a cardiac surgery program is supported in part by the revenue from angioplasties; the profitability of a cardiac surgery program, therefore, is enhanced and the break-even point is reduced. When angioplasty can be performed in the same institution without surgery, the financial viability of CV surgery must be reexamined. Should profit margins on cardiac surgery continue to fall as a result of competition, it is not unreasonable to predict that certain smaller programs will divest themselves of the surgical capability. Also, those considering future entry into the market will face higher entry barriers.

A final technological trend to be considered is the 1989 decision by Medicare to reimburse facility fees for freestanding, nonhospital catheterization laboratories. Some states, such as California, tightly control such laboratories, whereas other states, such as Florida, do not. Freestanding catheterization laboratories were commonplace in Florida even before Medicare began reimbursing facility fees.

It can be anticipated in these unregulated states that more and more cardiologists will offer this technology in their offices. Joint venture restrictions currently under consideration will not govern laboratories owned entirely by a large cardiology group. This trend, together with mobile and modular catheterization laboratories, will soften the competitive position of many existing diagnostic catheterization programs as more catheterization laboratories become available. Profits and, perhaps more important, cardiologists' demand for efficient scheduling for diagnostic cases while therapeutic cases tie up hospital catheterization laboratories will drive the demand for these outpatient and physician-owned alternatives.

The Future: Some Projections

A number of predictions can be made regarding the future of cardiovascular services:

1. *Major centers will lose market share.* No longer will cardiac surgery and cardiac catheterization services be performed exclusively or predominantly in large volume at just a few institutions. Volume will continue to be important, but the number of procedures required for a large and successful program and the number of procedures

required for a high-quality program will decline. This assumes, of course, that payer structures do not force more centralization among providers.

2. *Cardiovascular services will become staple services.* Because of the cardiovascular "food chain," that is, the relationship among referrals for primary care, subspecialty care, cardiology, diagnostic catheterization, therapeutic catheterization, and cardiac surgery, hospital management will see that cardiovascular services are necessary to sustain reasonable market share in primary care and general medical/surgical business.

3. *Price consolidation and stabilization will increase.* Market differences are substantial between low-cost providers and high-cost providers, although in some markets these differences have been minimized. Projected overall increases in competition will minimize the difference between low-cost and high-cost providers, exert a continuing downward pressure on the average case cost, and, ultimately, stabilize case costs for CV procedures. These factors will force CV programs to control operating costs more aggressively; failure to do so will have disastrous consequences.

4. *Expansion and consolidation will continue.* Relatively few programs offered cardiac surgery in the past, but that number will accelerate until the linkage between the interventional cardiac catheterization laboratory and the cardiac surgery suite is broken through technological developments, regulatory changes, standards of practice, or procedural innovations. Once that link is broken, it is conceivable that a consolidation in the market will occur. Those hospitals emerging as dominant players will not be the same ones that dominated in the past. This will occur as the result of demographic shifts and delivery system changes that result from the retirement of prominent older cardiovascular physicians and the emergence of new medical leadership.

5. *Use rates will stabilize.* Major shifts in usage rates are predicted for cardiac surgery, therapeutic catheterization, and diagnostic catheterization, although no conclusive evidence suggests that these rates will increase or decrease significantly over time. The most reasonable conclusion is that use rates experienced in mature markets will remain substantially the same.

6. *Technological innovation will flourish.* Considerable technological and procedural innovation has marked the recent past. The future will see continued progress in a number of areas, including therapeutic catheterization. No significant developments that will alter service delivery appear imminent, however. Although technological innovations occur quickly, the changes in the delivery system occur gradually.

Cardiovascular Services as a Maturing Market

The trends, assumptions, and predictions sketched in the preceding section suggest a dynamic and, in many respects, a turbulent future for cardiovascular services. Analyzing these services in the context of product life cycle theory may be helpful in anticipating future change.

Product life cycle analysis suggests that cardiovascular services, like inpatient services in general, are in transition from being a late growth market to becoming a mature market. As shown in figure 2-2, markets in transition tend to exhibit certain common characteristics. For example, in late growth markets it is important to know a product's cost and to control its quality, both achieved by *monitoring*.

Figure 2-2. The Product Life Cycle

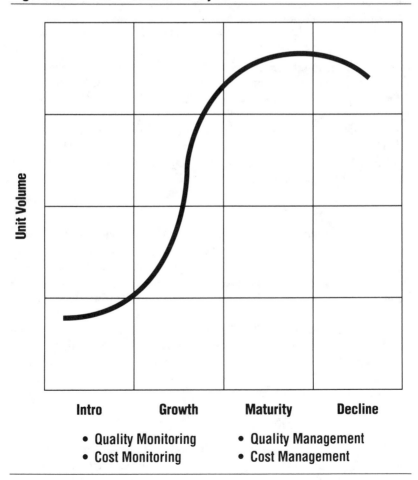

	Intro	Growth	Maturity	Decline

- Quality Monitoring   • Quality Management
- Cost Monitoring   • Cost Management

However, future CV programs will need to compete on the basis of quality and cost *management* — a subtle but essential difference. Knowing costs and controlling quality are much more passive than managing cost *and* quality. For example, a mature market with steady competitors and stable demand places increased pressure on pricing, requiring much innovation in managing costs.

Therefore, quality and cost will be predominant themes in subsequent chapters, as will the role of the physician in program management and development. This is because the physician plays the key role in managing both cost and quality.

The lessons to be learned from observing other industries and other services that have passed from a late growth market to a mature market suggest a need to redefine success in cardiovascular services. For example, past CV programs attempted to develop referral patterns that resulted in significant referrals and in-migration of patients from outside the traditional service area. However, in the future successful cardiovascular programs must ensure that patients who already use the hospital and those who are within the traditional program market area are treated in the hospital and not lost to outside competitors.

Hospitals will be challenged continually to redefine success in their markets and to question the assumptions that drove strategic planning and marketing in the past. In terms of competition, the emphasis will need to focus on managing *subtle differences* because major *qualitative differences* among competitors no longer will be a measure of competitive advantage.

Common pitfalls affect any market in transition from late growth to maturity. Some of them, which hamper participants in the cardiovascular market, are briefly described in the following sections, along with the "new reality," on how to avoid them.

Outdated Perceptions

Conventional wisdom among participants in cardiovascular services, principally those associated with large heart institutes and university centers, has held that cardiovascular services must be performed in volume to ensure high quality and competitive costs. The emerging reality is that quality outcomes for routine cases can be achieved at volumes significantly lower than the minimum standard of 200 cardiovascular surgery cases per year, a standard set during the late 1980s. The exact number that generates a sustainable level of quality will vary from site to site and from time to time according to the skill of the physicians involved, their involvement in other activities, case selection, and other factors. Nevertheless, the use of minimum volume thresholds is declining.

Quality As an Excuse

Leaders in growth markets often hide behind quality as an excuse for insisting that they continue as market headliners. Conventional wisdom holds that quality is key and can be ensured only in the large-volume programs that dominate the growth market.

The emerging realities are that in lower-volume programs acceptable quality outcomes for routine cases are quite attainable; further, quality differences are both understandable and predictable. For example, when a program is run by highly competent physicians, a high-quality program will emerge virtually without regard to volume, as is true with any clinical program. Conversely, mediocre physicians will create a low-quality program. These realities are true *regardless of volume*. Admittedly oversimplified, the point here is that the physician's role as it relates to program quality should not be underestimated. Quality is manageable when the real elements of quality are understood.

Reliance on New Initiatives and Products

Established providers grappling with loss of market share base their planning strategies on developing new products and initiatives. However, the reality in the health care marketplace suggests maintaining a focus on the staples, or the *basics,* of a program, product, or service. These basics include providing high-quality service, achieving a competitive pricing structure, ensuring convenience for patients and other customers, and providing appropriate and accurate information to the market regarding availability of the service.

Avoidance of Aggressive Sales for Some Programs

Conventional wisdom holds that low-volume cardiovascular services cannot be sold successfully and that smaller programs cannot achieve the highest levels of quality. However, the new reality is that only a small percentage of CV patients can benefit from the level of quality provided at a true center of excellence and by a master physician. Most patients in a mature clinical service are well tended by the physicians available within their own communities.

This provides an opportunity for smaller programs to become involved in aggressive sales based on successfully managing relationships with referring physicians, payers, and patients. It also requires larger programs to sell aggressively to maintain their market shares.

Strategic Program Elements

As hospitals consider their strategic options for cardiovascular services in the 1990s, there appear to be six generic elements around which successful strategies can be built:

- Delivery system
- Medical staff
- Physician leadership
- Quality
- Price and cost
- Competitors

These elements, summarized in figure 2-3 and discussed below, are major themes throughout the rest of the book.

Delivery System

To position its program, a hospital must examine the local and regional environments, where a variety of variables must be evaluated: major payers, aggregation and supply of physicians, utilization patterns, competition, historical referral and practice patterns, role of primary care physicians in the diagnosis and management of patients with cardiac disease, and so on. All are components of the hospital delivery system. Every community's delivery system is unique, and understanding how the delivery system functions is essential to the crafting of environmentally relevant strategy.

The delivery system will contain opportunities for, as well as obstacles to, strategic development. Delivery system components, including physician resources, other hospitals, access to other human resources, the role of managed care, local demographics, and so on, will significantly influence the strategic options for program development. Further, the efforts under way within this local delivery system to enhance regionalization or to

Figure 2-3. Strategic Program Elements

Delivery System: • Regionalization • Technology Dispersion • Exploit Technology/ Service Gaps	Quality: • Hospital • Physician • Team
Medical Staff: • Increasing Exclusivity • Increasing Inclusivity • Physician Star	Price and Cost: • Force Issue • Discourage Contracting • Address Physician Behavior
Physician Leadership: • Cardiologists • CV Surgeon • Unique Competencies	Competitors: • Affiliate • Keep Out • Develop Markets

encourage technology dissemination will be significant factors for consideration.

Medical Staff

Although facilities, technology, technical support personnel, and marketing campaigns have a definite impact on the success of clinical programs, *high-quality programs are built around competent physicians.* Therefore, considerable attention must be paid to the availability of cardiologists, cardiac surgeons, cardiac anesthesiologists, and other support physicians (pulmonologists, nephrologists, and infectious disease physicians, for example).

Because physicians are the single most important determinant of quality and cost, hospitals must build medical staffs that promote high-quality management and cost-effectiveness. Inevitably this will lead to a more exclusive medical staff, which, although contrary to the value systems of many hospital medical staffs, is a necessary step as competition in CV services intensifies and as hospitals compete increasingly on the basis of quality and cost. If physicians are understood to be distributors of hospital services — insofar as many hospital services cannot be distributed without the licensed physician "broker" — then hospitals will be obligated to consider alternative distribution strategies from the intensive distribution strategies employed in the past (as discussed later in this chapter).

Physician Leadership

When it comes to ensuring the success of cardiovascular programs, building a top-notch medical staff is not enough. The promotion of physician leadership is also essential. Conventional medical staff organization is democratic and egalitarian, and in many (though not all) settings this tradition has been effective. However, because new programs, programs in competitive markets, and programs with declining market shares all require change, they will benefit generally from a more authoritarian structure. In these situations, change is best facilitated through strong physician leadership.

Change increases an organization's need to make decisions, and these decisions become more frequent and more complex. In addition, the effects of these decisions on the medical staff can be very significant. The principal ingredient of a successful decision is a clear understanding of the decision's intent, that is, the objective or goal. To the extent the physician leader can clarify the goal and engineer goal congruity within the medical staff, the decision making will be more successful and the organization more effective.

Leadership is essential from the cardiology staff as well as within cardiovascular surgery. Defined leadership is also required in larger programs from cardiac anesthesiologists and pulmonologists/intensivists. Finally, a structure for leadership must be developed among these sections of the medical staff in order to facilitate goal formation, objective setting, and decision making.

Quality

As quality becomes a central theme in cardiovascular services, efforts to quantify or measure it will continue. At the same time, as cardiovascular services become more routine, the definition of quality will include non-clinical factors such as convenience and service delivery as well as the conventional morbidity-related and mortality-related measures.

This redefinition of quality is surprising given the current dialogue in clinical circles concerning appropriateness of care, mortality and morbidity rates, and efforts to measure and monitor quality. These factors will continue to be important, but the number of hospitals that offer acceptable clinical quality will increase. This redefinition will not make competing on the basis of quality easier, only more difficult by increasing the facets of quality to be considered in the marketing mix.

Price and Cost

Increased competition coupled with the growing influence of managed care in the cardiovascular market will continue to make price and cost major issues. As standard treatment protocols (discussed below) begin to replicate the practices of large-volume, low-cost programs and become commonplace even in community hospitals, the cost of cardiac surgery will become more uniform in given markets.

Competitors

The number of competitors in most markets will continue to increase. As mentioned earlier, the growth in cardiovascular services was fueled by the linkage between the catheterization laboratory and the cardiac surgery suite caused by standard-of-practice demands and regulations that required cardiac surgery backup for therapeutic catheterization procedures. As angioplasty techniques mature, it is logical to expect that the need for in-hospital cardiac surgery standby facilities will diminish. Whereas some may oppose this as unsafe, others strongly encourage it. Although the history of technological evolution clearly supports this prediction, the "how" and "when" are not yet understood. Furthermore, because competition and market size will not increase at the same rate, the number of procedures done by the typical program will continue to decline.

Once hospitals grasp these six program elements, they will have established the foundation of strategy development for a successful cardiovascular specialty program.

Physicians as Distributors

Many hospital services cannot be sold directly by the hospital to the patient; instead they are "sold" via physician referrals. This situation is roughly analogous to a producer's use of distributors to market its product to consumers, with physicians as the distributors of the health care "product." Extending this analogy may be a useful means of examining the role of physicians in a hospital's marketing strategy for CV services.

Marketing theory identifies three types of distribution strategies: intensive, selective, and exclusive. *Intensive* distribution strategies rely on sheer numbers of distributors to penetrate a market, with little regard to qualifications or credentials. *Selective* distribution places severe restrictions as to the number and quality of distributors. *Exclusive* distribution strategies, however, rely on the quality of a limited number of distributors who are expected to add value to the product.

Intensive distribution strategies in manufacturing industries are best utilized for low-cost and simple products to which the distributor adds no value. Chewing gum is an example of a product for which intensive distribution is appropriate. Hospitals historically have used the intensive distribution theory on the assumption that the more physicians the hospital has to distribute its services, the more services the hospital will sell. In the spectrum of hospital services, primary care services (such as those offered by family practitioners, general practitioners, and general internists) are considerably "simpler" than cardiovascular services. It is reasonable to predict that services related to primary care will continue to follow an intensive distribution strategy; that is, hospitals will attempt to secure relationships with as many primary care physicians as possible and thereby increase the volume of such services as routine laboratory and other diagnostic procedures.

As a product increases in value and complexity, a nondiscriminating strategy becomes increasingly inappropriate for the producer. The distributor's role in adding value to the product becomes critical to the producer's ability to market and sell its goods or services. For example, Levi jeans are sold through selected retailers on the basis of the value added by the retailer's reputation. Automobiles are sold through exclusive distributor relationships because of the value that the dealer adds to the sale of the car. Note also that the more restricted the delivery channel, the more the interest of the distributor (physician) parallels that of the producer (hospital).

This principle also applies to cardiovascular services, a product whose value is enhanced by virtue of the quality of the physician–patient relationship in the delivery of CV services. Cardiology services are apt to be distributed increasingly on a selective basis, whereas cardiac surgery will move to *exclusive distribution* relationships in which hospitals develop exclusive contracts with a single group of cardiac surgeons.

This evolution of distribution strategy is in keeping with our understanding of CV services moving from late growth to mature markets in which providers will compete increasingly on the basis of quality and cost. To do so successfully, medical staffs must be structured not simply on the number of licensed physicians but on the quality and cost-effectiveness of each physician/distributor. Current and future market forces will likely result in more stringent privileging requirements, including economic performance indicators.

Standard Treatment Protocols

The skills of physicians coupled with their unique practice patterns are the principal variables in (severity-adjusted) case costs. Large-volume, low-cost cardiovascular programs have built their success around highly skilled physicians who have developed efficient practice patterns. These practice patterns become the standard of practice for those programs, and other physicians are encouraged, expected, and even required to follow these patterns. The resulting *standard treatment protocols* (STPs) ensure the success of the cardiovascular program. Smaller programs without the benefit of such physician leadership must devise these STPs and ensure that physicians have incentives to use them.

Note from table 2-7 that total volume and case price do not correlate positively. Institutional size and prestige also correlate poorly with case price, because many of the largest institutions in the state may be among the most costly. Although poor correlation may seem reasonably attributable to case severity distribution, such an explanation does not allow for the fact that several of these large centers are the best known, include heart centers that show the highest volume, and consistently are among the most efficient providers. The clear message is that case costs can be managed effectively even at annual volumes lower than 200 cases. To do so requires modifying physician practice patterns through methods such as STPs (a process described further in chapter 4).

Summary

In a field changing as rapidly as cardiovascular services, hospital managers need to have access to a great deal of information, anticipate change, predict as accurately as possible long-term trends in the marketplace, and react appropriately. This chapter examined a number of factors that affect the market, covering successful strategies for avoiding pitfalls. A summary of these key points includes the following observations:

- Technological innovations will continue to have an impact in both invasive and noninvasive cardiology.
- Prices for CV services will decline further and then stabilize.
- Flat-use rates for various procedures should be assumed for program planning.
- Cardiovascular programs will continue to disperse into previously unserved or underserved areas.
- Cardiovascular surgery programs will expand until standby is no longer required for PTCA cases.
- Competition will increase substantially.
- Providers will need to compete on the basis of quality and cost.
- Providers should focus on improving basic program elements.
- Physician distributors will be central to the success of any program.
- Standard treatment protocols will make providers more competitive.

☐ Reference

1. National Association of Manufacturers. Meeting the health care crisis. *Medical Benefits* 6(12):1-2, June 30, 1989.

Chapter 3

Local Market Assessment

Planning for a cardiovascular program — whether for introducing a new cardiovascular service, expanding existing services, or repositioning an an existing program — must be based on a thorough assessment of the market. All planning and development must be *market-driven,* which means the nature, size, and characteristics of the target markets for specific programs and services must determine how those services are structured and delivered. Moreover, only the realities of the marketplace can accurately predict successful strategies.

All too often, however, hospital planners and administrators fail to perform a thorough and complete critical analysis of the marketplace. Rather than basing their planning perspective on external factors (such as market area, market share, and demographics) — or moving from *outside in,* planners are overly influenced by internal factors (such as the wishes, intuition, or response to political pressure of management) — thus planning from *inside out.* Misjudging the market carries serious, potentially fatal, consequences for any hospital program, cardiovascular programs included. The financial and political risks that accompany the failure of a program or service are simply too costly to allow an organization to forgo a thorough understanding of marketplace phenomena.

This chapter focuses on the critical steps involved in assessing the *external* market. The chapter begins with an overview of the process and then details the types and sources of data required and the analytical methodology used to refine the data into information useful for planning program development. A method is presented for competitor analysis, along with a framework for assessing critical forces in the competitive environment. Information essential to an assessment is highlighted here. Subsequent chapters provide in-depth discussions of the methodologies for translating market factors uncovered in the assessment into specific plans of action.

The Market Assessment Process

Assessing the market for cardiovascular services can be accomplished by a variety of processes. One process is outlined in figure 3-1, a checklist of elements included in that process.

Note that often the market assessment process is a prelude to preparing a strategic marketing plan or a business plan. The process illustrated in figure 3-1 can be expanded or abbreviated on the basis of the requirements of the planning effort. Market assessment comprises four major planning steps:

1. Prestudy
2. Data collection and analysis
3. Determination of findings
4. Development of conclusions and recommendations

Step 1: Prestudy

As in any decision-making process, objectives must be outlined. Prestudy calls for the formulation and formalization of objectives, problems, and opportunities to be addressed through the assessment process.

Prestudy must also consider the physical constraints on program development. For example, if objectives included researching the potential for a new cardiac catheterization laboratory, the planner could note that space is already strained by existing cardiac services and identify overcrowding as a possible problem to be addressed in the assessment. Available space in a medical office building on the hospital campus may be an opportunity for a catheterization laboratory location. In most studies, it will be critical to integrate the research effort within the context of organizationwide space design planning and physical facility development.

Resources required for implementing the planning effort also must be assessed accurately. These might include significant staff time, consulting assistance, formation of a planning task force (which may include members of the medical staff), allocation of funds for the purchase of data, and so on.

Once the objectives, the problems and opportunities, and the support necessary to complete the process have been identified, a *work plan* can be completed. This work plan, which can be simple or elaborate depending on the scope of the project, must state the following: project objectives, resources required, participants, appropriate reporting relationships, delineation of responsibility and authority, description of the final project, and projected time frame for project completion.

Step 2: Data Collection and Analysis

Based on conclusions drawn during the prestudy phase, data collection can begin. Data collection will require definition of data elements and determination

Figure 3-1. CV Program Assessment and Strategic Planning Process

Prestudy

- State objectives
- Identify problems and opportunities
- Integrate with space design planning/physical facility development
- Develop work plan
- Establish time frame
- State resources required
- Identify reporting relationships

Data Collection and Analysis

Data definitions (primary and secondary sources):
- Define requirements (category, level of detail, time period, and so forth)
- Specify services (department, service, person, system)
- Identify limitations and weaknesses

Data collection process:
- Specify data-processing requirements
- Specify format/reformat requirements (preliminary and final)
- Specify computerization requirements for collection and analysis
- Prepare preliminary management report and summary

External Environmental Analysis

Market share:
- Define market area(s)
- Define product line by DRG
- Define other data parameters (age, sex, payer source, and so forth)
- Obtain hospital discharge data through state planning agency
- Prepare summary and conclusions

Market area demographics:
- Define data parameters (age cohorts, sex, population, income, and so forth)
- Obtain current-year estimates, appropriate-year projections
- Match demographic data with market share data
- Prepare summary and conclusions

Competitors:
- Identify key competitors (overall and/or by product line)
- Identify competitive SWOTs (strengths/weaknesses/opportunities/threats)
- Determine overall competitive advantage/strategy
- Identify significant referral patterns
- Assess impact on existing/proposed program/service on key competitors (offensive/defensive response)
- Prepare summary and conclusions

Usage rates (use, frequency, and prevalence):
- Define categories (clinical and age/sex cohorts)
- Model actual usage rates via computer
- Summarize actual usage rates by age/sex cohorts, by market area
- Prepare summary and conclusions

(Continued on next page)

Figure 3-1. (Continued)

Projected usage rates by market area:
• Project usage rates based on historical and projected use and population projections
• Model projected usage rates by service or market area via computer
• Prepare summary and conclusions

Specialized Market Research (if Requested)

• Define required primary research
• Define research goal and objectives
• Specify research methodology
• Establish time frames and budget
• Implement research plan
• Tabulate results via computer
• Prepare analysis, summary, and conclusions

Internal Environmental Analysis

Existing cardiovascular services:
• Research background and history
• Describe current services and resources
  —Noninvasive cardiology department
  —Cardiac catheterization laboratory
  —Cardiovascular surgery
  —Critical care nursing services
  —Cardiac rehabilitation program
  —Standing committees related to cardiovascular services program
• Identify cardiovascular services-related quality assurance and standards programs
• Identify existing patient education programs
• Identify current postdischarge programs
• Review pricing and contracting structure

Department operating reports (revenue and expense reports, by month, for the past two years)

Cardiac service statistics (by month, by physician—segregated by inpatient and outpatient data for the past two years)

Cardiovascular market share by patient origin

Review of associated departments:
• Radiology
• Clinical laboratory
• Respiratory care
• Physical therapy
• Pharmacy
• Emergency department

Medical staff information:
• Obtain physician roster
• Develop profile of physicians (number, age, board certification, and so on, by specialty)
• Summarize physician activity (referrals, procedures, patient days, and so on)
• Describe significant referral patterns
• Define role of physicians in program
• Define role of hospital-based physicians

Figure 3-1. (Continued)

Interviews

- Select interview candidates on the basis of their relevance to assessment
- Determine interview questions
- Conduct interviews
- Prepare summary and conclusions

Determination of Findings

Market area:
- Define market area
- Chart market area population trends
- Chart market area usage rates (actual and projected)

Market share:
- Display share by competitor and market area
- Graph market share trends over selected time periods

SWOT programs and services analysis:
- Prepare SWOT for program/service
- Prepare SWOT for related and/or supportive departments and those on which program/service will have an impact

Competitors:
- Summarize the key competitor analysis (key characteristics, market position strategies, strengths and weaknesses)
- Assess likely offensive and defensive strategies

Overall data summary and conclusions

Development of Conclusions and Recommendations

Note: Conclusions will be directly influenced by, and will include a discussion of, the following key factors: markets, products, services, market "niches," pricing/packaging, medical staff development, equipment and facilities, product line management, and facility-specific operations optimization.

Strategy formulation:
- Identify significant strategic opportunities and threats
- Analyze current goals and suggest necessary revision of goals
- Provide preliminary estimates of financial, operational, strategic, and political feasibility
- Formulate strategy and strategic decision-making process

Objective setting:
- Set objectives based on strategy formulation and revised goals

Recommendations:
- Based on complete analysis of information, propose recommendations matched with strategy, goals, and objectives
- Recommend strategies
- Identify principal barriers
- Recommend tactics
- Identify major gateways
- Recommend resource requirements

Implementation plan:
- Define how recommended actions will be implemented (by whom, by what date, with what resources, for what expected outcomes)
- Identify implications of program implementation
- Set out evaluation mechanism to monitor implementation
- Define feedback loops to implement changes in plans as required by internal and external conditions

of optimal data sources. Data elements to be defined include, but are not limited to, the following:

- Description of primary and secondary service areas
- Description of cardiovascular service area
- Demographics for counties, zip codes, census tracts, or health facility planning areas included in service areas
- Available information on area competitors
- Available information on physicians in community
- Assessments of medical staff activity levels
- State and local volumes for cardiovascular services including cardiac surgery, cardiac catheterization, and angioplasty
- Financial reports for the cardiovascular product line

These data elements will form the baseline of materials necessary to begin market analysis. Additional data will be identified as step 2 is completed and will depend on the scope of the project planned. The data collection process includes specification of data formats, determination of data-processing requirements, and assessment of computer capabilities for data collection and analysis. Data definitions and the data collection process should then be summarized in a preliminary management report.

As mentioned earlier, the market (or the environment) generally is seen to encompass external and internal forces. Both must be accounted for accurately in assessing the market. Because the external environment usually is the larger issue under consideration, most of this chapter will be devoted to those methods that define the external market geographically, quantify the market through usage rate calculations, assess market size, compute market share, anticipate competitor reaction, and so on.

Assessing the internal environment can be a complex process, and the outline of the internal environment components in figure 3-1 focuses primarily on quantitative data elements. It should be understood, however, that the *qualitative* aspects of the internal environment — such as the relationships among the medical staff, political struggles within the management staff, concern over preserving the status quo, and so on — are often of greater importance than the quantitative measures. Interviews thus become an essential component of the assessment and planning process inasmuch as the interview process is the principal method for gathering qualitative and subjective data.

Interviews should be conducted with members of both the internal and external markets. These interviews will involve physicians (including those *not* on the medical staff) and management personnel but may also encompass community leaders, board members, former patients, and members of the community at large. The interview process may be formal, such as programmed personal interviews with specific predetermined questions; telephone interviews, performed as part of a market research process; focus groups; unstructured personal interviews; or questionnaire interviews.

Interview information can be invaluable to the management team in gauging the internal and external markets and identifying key emerging trends or attitudes. For example, political mood swings within the medical community, information concerning competitors (other hospitals), or reports regarding activities of physicians or medical groups in the market can be useful indicators.

The interview process should also be used as a communications link to the community, particularly the medical community. Asking physicians for their input is a simple but vital step in managing physician relations, one that often is overlooked.

Step 3: Determination of Findings

Once gathered and analyzed by management staff and the designated work group, the data will be drafted into a series of findings, which are factual statements summarizing the analyzed data. The findings will include a description of the market area, calculation of market share, a description of market area competitors, and so on (discussed in the section on external market assessment). Also, based on interviews, they could include subjective factors.

Step 4: Development of Conclusions and Recommendations

Depending on the objectives arrived at in step 1, the final step of the market assessment may be a management report briefly listing quantitative findings such as the usage rates for cardiovascular procedures (usually reported as a rate per 1,000 population per year) and a calculation of the size of the market based on these current usage rate figures. This report may be the preliminary step for a larger project such as developing a marketing plan for an existing cardiovascular program or a strategic plan for the addition of a new or expanded cardiovascular service.

The final product of the market assessment process may also be an expanded analytical report, complete with conclusions drawn from the factual findings. Conclusions will include forecasts of future directions within the market; actions to be expected from competitors; preliminary estimates of financial, operational, strategic, and political feasibility; projections of resources required; and so forth. These conclusions in turn will lead to development of specific recommendations, including an initial outline of strategy issues. Recommendations will be based on identified market trends and directions and will focus on such areas as program development, new markets and services, medical staff development, pricing, and packaging of services. Although recommendations can be addressed in depth in a strategic plan or business plan (the specific focus of chapters 4 through 6), often the market assessment is expanded to become a part of that larger process.

To the extent that the market assessment includes recommendations, it should also suggest an implementation plan. Implementation should be addressed at least in terms of what the next steps in the process will be, assignment of responsibilities, and the schedule for implementation.

External Assessment

To conduct an external market assessment for a cardiovascular services program, a hospital should examine at least seven factors that influence the market:

1. Market area
2. Service area demographics
3. Market share
4. Inpatient and outpatient data
5. Usage rate projections
6. Current referral volume
7. Competitor analysis

Market Area

In evaluating an external market, its geographic service boundaries must be known so that the market area can be characterized and statistically analyzed. Hospitals typically will have predefined market or service areas based on patient origin studies or other market analyses already available. Some of these sources will have defined each product line or service separately, whereas others will have utilized a single market area for the entire mix of patients seen.

If market area information is not already available, it can be developed by analyzing the hospital's patient demographic data. These data may include number of patients by zip codes, census tracts, or other common geographical measures of patient origin.

Depending on the specific product line under consideration, it is not uncommon for market areas to vary in size of potential market share (discussed later in this chapter). By analyzing patient origin for cardiovascular services *specifically,* planners can acquire product-specific information that will help determine whether they can capture a wider potential market than would hold true for other services. For example, because invasive cardiology historically has been considered more tertiary in nature than general surgery, patients will be referred to the hospital from a wider geographic area than is typical for other services. Although analysis of a specific patient population is easier for hospitals with existing cardiovascular services, the analysis of patients receiving cardiovascular services available through other data bases can be extremely helpful in program planning.

Once an overall market area is defined, it may be helpful to further segregate the area into more refined boundaries of hospital influence, or market share. The *primary* market area is typically considered the region from which a substantial majority—generally 75 percent—of the hospital's patients come. The *secondary* market area is determined by identifying those areas that will bring the cumulative patient total to 90 percent, or an additional 15 percent. The remaining areas constitute the tertiary market area.

The geographic size of the market that a hospital will designate for planning purposes will depend on many factors, including the presence of competitors, historical referral patterns, natural boundaries, barriers to access, and so forth.

Service Area Demographics

Once geographic market areas have been identified and formalized, area demographics should be analyzed. Sources for this information include local governments, planning agencies, and commercial data companies. Depending on the unique characteristics of the market in question, geographic subunits for analysis will vary; these subunits may be zip codes, census tracts, health facility planning areas, or counties. Generally, the hospital's planning department will have determined subunits beforehand.

Data required to assess the market for CV services will include population size within each geographic subunit, including age and sex cohorts. Because cardiovascular disease is related to demographic factors such as age, sex, and race, these three factors are important to study as part of demographic analysis. Projections of changes in these categories for the next three to five years are helpful and customarily available. Incidence rates for specific DRG (diagnosis-related group) procedures can be calculated by age and sex cohorts in certain areas. These incidence rates can be especially helpful in forecasting the market size of smaller geographic areas such as specific zip codes and targeting Medicare market volumes by geographic area. Where information on projected changes is unavailable, data similar to those provided in table 3-1 should be developed and utilized.

Because the incidence of heart disease increases with age, more refined projections will take into account the age and sex cohorts of the population and the varying incidence and use rates that will result when this information is obtainable.

Market Share

Market share analysis is an important consideration in evaluations of the size and characteristics of a cardiovascular services market. *Market share* is simply a hospital's percentage (actual or potential) of the total market for a specific diagnostic category or procedure in a specific market area for a specific time period. Determining market share also helps in analyzing competition.

Table 3-1. Demographic Analysis of Sample Hospital's Service Area

	1980 Population		1986 Estimate		1991 Projection	
Population	150,489		166,598		202,646	
In group quarters	4,188		4,826		6,053	
Households	64,183		72,422		88,921	
One person	23,170	36.1%	26,506	36.6%	32,901	37.0%
Two persons	20,923	32.6%	26,506	32.2%	32,901	31.9%
Three to four persons	14,890	23.2%	17,521	24.2%	22,141	24.9%
Over five persons	5,198	8.1%	4,997	6.9%	5,424	6.1%
Average household size		2.28		2.23		2.21
Families	35,816		38,614		46,608	
Race						
White	122,498	81.4%	128,614	77.2%	149,958	74.0%
Hispanic	21,369	14.2%	29,988	18.0%	45,595	22.5%
Black	16,102	10.7%	21,325	12.8%	29,789	14.7%
American Indian	1,203	0.8%	1,667	1.0%	4,256	2.1%
Asian/Pacific Islander	8,578	5.7%	11,828	7.1%	16,414	8.1%
Other	2,257	1.5%	3,165	1.9%	4,255	2.1%
Age						
0 to 5	12,039	8.0%	14,994	9.0%	19,049	9.4%
6 to 13	13,845	9.2%	14,327	8.6%	19,251	9.5%
14 to 17	7,524	5.0%	6,997	4.2%	7,093	3.5%
18 to 20	7,825	5.2%	6,831	4.1%	7,701	3.8%
21 to 24	13,394	8.9%	13,161	7.9%	13,172	6.5%
25 to 34	23,593	19.0%	36,152	21.7%	44,177	21.8%
35 to 44	15,199	10.1%	20,991	12.6%	29,181	14.4%
45 to 54	13,995	9.3%	12,495	7.5%	15,604	7.7%
55 to 64	16,403	10.9%	16,826	10.1%	18,035	8.9%
65+	21,670	14.4%	23,824	14.3%	29,181	14.4%
Median age		31.8		32.4		32.9
Males	73,174		82,413		101,093	
0 to 20	20,708	28.3%	21,839	26.5%	26,891	26.6%
21 to 44	29,709	40.6%	37,086	45.0%	46,098	45.6%
45 to 64	14,708	20.1%	14,422	17.5%	16,883	16.7%
65+	8,047	11.0%	9,065	11.0%	11,322	11.2%
Females	77,315		84,185		101,553	
0 to 20	20,566	26.6%	21,467	25.5%	26,302	25.9%
21 to 44	27,370	35.4%	33,169	39.4%	40,621	40.0%
45 to 64	15,695	20.3%	14,817	17.6%	16,756	16.5%
65+	16,607	17.6%	14,817	17.6%	17,978	17.7%

Source: AHA Hospital Technology Series, includes *Executive Briefing, Technology Scanner, and Guide-line Report* 1988, American Hospital Association, Division of Clinical Services and Technology.

Market share information can be developed to indicate overall market size and distribution by hospital facility in terms of patient discharges, average lengths of stay, payer sources, age and sex cohorts, and other such characteristics.

Because of increasing emphasis on cardiovascular case prices, case price information should also be gathered and evaluated by market share. Aggregating these data for the market area under study will help define further the market and the competitors within that market.

Generally, calculations of market share information can be obtained from state planning agencies, commercial data companies, regional cooperative data collection agencies, or other sources. These data may even be available by *ICD-9-CM* codes, DRGs, or aggregated by product line. Although less exact because of their aggregate nature, DRG data usually are more readily available and simpler to analyze. Also, DRG data are often also available via the hospital's patient accounts or medical record department, resulting in an opportunity to compare charges for similar types of cases.

Depending on the nature of the targeted procedures or diagnoses, research needs may require that patients be analyzed by more finite definitions than can be achieved with DRGs. This would be the case when planning programs to address specific cardiac conditions. For example, if hospital management wanted to study rates for percutaneous transluminal coronary angioplasty (PTCA), it is only one of the many procedures included in DRG 112: percutaneous cardiovascular procedures. Therefore, it may be more appropriate to determine whether data are available for PTCA through the use of *ICD-9-CM* procedure codes 36.01, 36.02, and 36.05, and to study these results.

The level of detail required in any market share analysis will be a function of the availability of reliable current information, the nature of the investment under consideration, and the degree of risk associated with that investment. For example, the risk of entry or expansion in a market typically is related to the presence and type of competition in that market.

The timeliness of data can be a problem: Even if market data are six months to several years old, they still must be used when no newer data can be identified. If the detailed data base is more than several years old, efforts should be made to gather recent *anecdotal* information, which will help in identifying significant changes. For example, competitor hospitals may have reported catheterization volumes or cardiac surgery volumes to a certain agency (or agencies), or data may be obtainable through direct contact or discussion with the hospitals' medical staff.

The expanded data-reporting capabilities of many states (such as California, Florida, and Colorado) will provide an important planning data base for hospitals. Because the information gathered by state and federal governmental agencies is in the public domain, a large body of market and competitor data is available, particularly with respect to the market for inpatient services.

Examples of the information needed for planning cardiovascular services can be found in tables 3-2 through 3-4. Where local or regional statewide

Table 3-2. Market Share by Zip Code and Product Line, Antelope Valley Market Area

Hospital	Total Discharges	Total Days	Total Charges	Average Length of Stay	Average Charge per Day	Average Charge per Case	Market Share (%)
Cardiovascular—Medical							
Lancaster Community Hosp.	981	5,704	6,708,314	5.8	1,176.07	6,838.24	34.2
Antelope Valley Hosp. Med. Ctr.	946	6,034	5,642,037	6.4	935.04	5,964.10	33.0
Palmdale Hosp. Med. Ctr.	481	2,131	2,782,128	4.4	1,305.55	5,784.05	16.8
LA County High Desert Hosp.	167	1,524	996,650	9.1	653.97	5,967.96	5.8
Kaiser—Panorama City	88	510	0	5.8	0.00	0.00	3.1
All other hospitals	203	1,055	2,887	5.2	2.74	5,707.99	7.1
Total	2,866	18,958	17,287,851	5.9	1,019.45	6,032.05	100.0
Cardiovascular—Surgical							
Lancaster Community Hosp.	358	3,513	8,229,190	9.8	2,342.50	22,986.56	54.1
Antelope Valley Hosp. Med. Ctr.	90	1,125	1,655,529	12.5	1,471.58	18,394.77	13.6
Palmdale Hosp. Med. Ctr.	39	345	803,690	8.8	2,329.54	20,607.44	5.9
Kaiser—Panorama City	21	137	0	6.5	0.00	0.00	3.2
St. Vincent Med. Ctr.	20	187	385,800	9.3	2,063.10	19,290.00	3.0
LA County High Desert Hosp.	16	191	159,943	11.9	837.40	9,996.44	2.4
Kaiser—Los Angeles	12	95	0	7.9	0.00	0.00	1.8
Encino Hosp.	10	76	291,232	7.6	3,832.00	29,123.20	1.5
Santa Barbara Cottage Hosp.	10	68	108,105	6.8	1,589.78	10,810.50	1.5
The Hospital of the Good Samaritan	9	89	180,881	9.9	2,032.37	20,097.89	1.4
Cedars Sinai Med Ctr.	8	109	337,918	13.6	3,100.17	42,239.75	1.2
UCLA Med. Ctr.	8	43	107,375	5.4	2,497.09	13,421.88	1.2
All other hospitals	61	657	80,244	10.8	122.14	17,133.41	9.2
Total	662	6,635	13,304,801	10.0	2,005.25	20,097.89	100.0
Cardiovascular—Total							
Lancaster Comm. Hosp.	1,339	9,217	14,937,504	6.9	1,620.65	11,155.72	38.0
Antelope Valley Hosp. Med. Ctr.	1,036	7,159	7,297,566	6.9	1,019.36	7,043.98	29.4
Palmdale Hosp. Med. Ctr.	520	2,476	3,585,818	4.8	1,448.23	6,895.80	14.7
LA County High Desert Hosp.	183	1,715	1,156,593	9.4	674.40	6,320.18	5.2
Kaiser—Panorama City	109	647	0	5.9	0.00	0.00	3.1
All other hospitals	341	2,379	3,615,171	7.0	1,519.62	10,601.67	9.7
Total	3,528	23,593	30,592,652	6.7	1,296.68	8,671.39	100.0

Source: AHA Hospital Technology Series, includes *Executive Briefing, Technology Scanner, and Guideline Report* 1988, American Association, Division of Clinical Services and Technology.

Table 3-3. Sample Community Hospital Cardiovascular Services Product Line Summary, Primary Market Area: FY 1986

Product Line	Total			Average			Market Share (%)			Financial Class (%)				Age 65+ (%)
	Total Discharges	Total Days	Total Charges	LOS	$/Day	$/Discharge	Discharges	Days	Charges	Medicare	MediCal	HMO/PPO	Others	
Medical	981	5,704	$ 6,708,314	5.8	$1,176	$ 6,838	34.2	29.7	38.8	43.8	5.3	5.4	21.7	56.3
Surgical	358	3,513	$ 8,229,190	9.8	$2,343	$22,987	54.1	52.9	61.9	50.8	3.6	3.6	41.9	48.3
Total	1,339	9,217	$14,937,504	6.9	$1,621	$11,156	38.0	39.1	48.8	57.4	4.9	4.9	32.9	54.1

Note: Pediatrics is included in all appropriate discharges.

Source: California Office of Statewide Health Planning and Development, 1988.

Table 3-4.   Financial Class Utilization of CV Services by Zip Code and Product Line

Hospital	Medicare Discharges	Medicare Days	Medicare ALOS	Average Medicare Charges	MediCal Discharges	MediCal Days
Medical						
Lancaster Community Hosp.	586	4,080	7.0	7,631	62	254
Antelope Valley Hosp. Med. Ctr.	542	4,292	7.9	7,028	31	178
Palmdale Hosp. Med. Ctr.	279	1,501	5.4	6,674	39	116
LA County High Desert Hosp.	36	516	14.3	6,833	67	737
Kaiser—Panorama City	41	271	6.6	0		
All other hospitals	84	538	6.4	6,989	13	64
Total	1,568	11,198	7.1	7,000	202	1,349
Surgical						
Lancaster Community Hosp.	182	1,898	10.4	22,247	13	119
Antelope Valley Hosp. Med. Ctr.	46	676	14.7	21,093	5	37
Palmdale Hosp. Med. Ctr.	33	304	9.2	21,249		
Kaiser—Panorama City	11	61	5.5	0		
St. Vincent Med. Ctr.	3	29	9.7	17,403	2	9
LA County High Desert Hosp.	3	50	16.7	15,591	7	71
Kaiser—Los Angeles	5	60	12.0	0		
Encino Hosp.	7	58	8.3	34,900		
Santa Barbara Cottage Hosp.	3	27	9.0	11,478		
The Hospital of the Good Samaritan	3	53	17.7	30,983		
Cedars Sinai Med. Ctr.	3	51	20.3	61,661		
UCLA Med. Ctr.						
All other hospitals	25	259	10.4	17,483	8	122
Total	324	3,536	10.9	21,028	35	358
Total						
Lancaster Community Hosp.	768	5,978	7.8	11,094	65	373
Antelope Valley Hosp. Med. Ctr.	588	4,968	8.4	8,128	36	215
Palmdale Hosp. Med. Ctr.	312	1,805	5.8	8,216	39	116
LA County High Desert Hosp.	39	566	14.5	7,507	74	808
Kaiser—Panorama City	52	332	6.4	0		
All other hospitals	133	1,085	8.2	12,279	23	195
Total	1,892	14,734	7.8	9,402	237	1,707

Source: AHA Hospital Technology Series, includes *Executive Briefing, Technology Scanner, and Guideline Report,* 1988, American Hospital Association, Division of Clinical Services and Technology.

				Medical					
MediCal ALOS	Average MediCal Charges	HMO/PHP Discharges	HMO/PHP Days	HMO/PHP ALOS	Average HMO/PHO Charges	Other Discharges	Other Days	Other ALOS	Average Other Charges
4.9	5,878	53	213	4.0	5,087	290	1,157	4.0	4,729
5.7	5,612	40	135	3.4	3,987	333	1,429	4.3	4,503
3.0	4,265	45	107	2.4	3,827	118	407	3.4	4,928
11.0	6,154	7	26	3.7	4,717	57	245	4.3	5,356
		47	239	5.1	0				
4.9	4,567	20	121	6.0	3,960	86	332	3.9	5,035
6.7	5,533	212	841	1.0	3,366	884	3,570	4.0	5,096

				Surgical					
9.2	22,695	13	89	6.8	15,814	150	1,407	9.4	24,531
7.4	16,395	2	10	5.0	10,157	37	402	10.9	15,756
		1	2	2.0	14,026	5	39	7.8	17,689
		10	76	7.6	0				
4.5	10,601	7	53	7.6	16,404	8	96	12.0	24,695
10.1	8,811					6	70	11.7	8,583
		7	35	5.0	0				
						3	18	6.0	
						7	41	5.9	10,524
		2	15	7.5	21,004	4	21	5.3	11,481
						5	48	9.6	30,587
		2	3	1.5	3,111	6	40	6.7	16,859
15.3	22,299	2	8	4.0	3,885	26	268	10.3	16,227
10.2	18,236	46	291	6.3	8,929	257	2,450	9.5	21,178

				Total					
5.7	9,242	66	302	4.6	7,200	440	2,564	5.8	12,139
6.0	7,109	42	145	3.5	4,281	370	1,831	4.9	5,628
3.0	4,265	46	109	2.5	4,049	123	446	3.6	5,447
10.9	6,406	7	26	3.7	4,717	63	315	5.0	5,663
		57	315	5.5	0				
8.5	11,259	40	235	5.9	6,251	145	864	6.0	10,159
7.2	7,409	258	1,132	4.4	4,358	1,141	6,020	5.3	8,697

data are not readily available, information from states with more sophisticated data collection capabilities may provide planning guidance. Such data contain length of stay, average charge, payer mix, and related information. Specifically, incidence rates from other states may be useful for inferring characteristics of the market in question. This level of detail may not substantially change the total market area projections, but it will assist in targeting cardiovascular patients by zip code or census tracts if the age-adjusted incidence rates are multiplied by the zip code population in each age cohort. Targeting patients by zip code in this fashion helps tailor marketing activities, allowing extra attention to be focused in the areas with high cardiovascular patient density.

Discharge data must be analyzed and summarized to extract the required information from the data base. For example, tables 3-3 and 3-4 aggregate and summarize data specific to the cardiovascular market. Table 3-5 displays the age distribution of patients discharged with a primary cardiovascular diagnosis by the zip code of their origin. Table 3-6 exhibits the market share captured by each of the top four hospitals for medical and surgical cardiovascular discharges. Finally, a determination is made of the incidence of discharges for medical and surgical cardiovascular diagnosis, and a use rate within the area under study is calculated.

By comparing the total incidence of a particular procedure for a specific geographic area and subtracting the actual services performed by hospitals in the service area, in-migration or out-migration of patients can be determined. If hospitals in the market area performed more open-heart surgeries than there are residents in the same area who received open-heart surgery, then patients are coming into the market, or "in-migrating," for open-heart surgery. Conversely, if hospitals in the market performed fewer open-heart surgeries than were performed on market area residents, then patients are leaving the market, or "out-migrating," for this procedure. Historically, urban centers have experienced in-migration due to patients who come in from suburban, semirural, and rural areas for open-heart surgery. In-migration and out-migration are important factors that can create statistical skewing of analytical results.

In the example used in table 3-7, the total number of discharged CV patients from the service area exceeded the number of CV patients discharged by the sample hospital. Thus, the area experienced a net out-migration of cardiac patients. It is projected that 498 patients from the service area will be discharged from hospitals outside the service area in the study year for cardiovascular conditions.

A number of other factors may affect potential market share, and a number of categories can be studied (severity of illness between programs is another example). Planners should determine these specific categories when studying the external market factors.

Table 3-5. Sample Community Hospital Patients Discharged, Age Distribution by Zip Code: 1988

Zip Code	Name	1988 Population	Age Distribution (%)										Median Age in 1988
			0-4	5-11	12-17	18-24	25-34	35-44	45-54	55-64	65-74	75+	
9xxxx	A	4,510	7.2	9.8	10.0	11.2	13.1	15.8	14.1	10.0	6.0	2.9	33.4
9xxxx	B	10,699	9.7	14.0	9.7	13.4	24.5	18.0	6.8	1.9	1.3	0.6	26.2
9xxxx	C	57,153	8.2	10.7	9.5	11.1	15.5	13.6	10.7	9.4	7.0	4.3	31.7
9xxxx	D	24,613	8.1	10.5	9.2	11.4	15.6	13.0	11.1	9.9	7.3	3.6	31.7
9xxxx	E	5,674	*	*	*	*	*	*	*	*	*	*	*
9xxxx	F	5,339	8.4	10.7	10.3	11.1	11.9	10.5	10.1	10.8	9.7	6.4	32.7
9xxxx	G	53,745	9.3	11.7	9.4	11.0	15.6	31.2	10.2	9.1	6.8	3.7	30.4
9xxxx	H	2,578	*	*	*	*	*	*	*	*	*	*	*
9xxxx	I	1,317	*	*	*	*	*	*	*	*	*	*	*

Note: An asterisk indicates that no information is available. Zip code information for age has not been updated. Small population figures will not affect totals.

Source: CACI Marketing Systems, Fairfax, Virginia, 1988.

Table 3-6. Sample Community Hospital Market Share Summary: Top Four Market Share Positions by Cardiovascular Services Product Line, Primary Market Area

Product Line	No. 1 Market Share		No. 2 Market Share		No. 3 Market Share		No. 4 Market Share		Total %	% All Other Hospitals
	Hospital	% Total Discharges	Hospital	% Total Discharges	Hospital	% Total Discharges	Hospital	% Total Discharges		
Medical	A	34.2	C	33.0	D	16.8	E	5.8	89.8	10.2
Surgical	A	54.1	C	13.6	D	5.9	B	3.2	76.8	23.2
Total	A	38.0	C	29.4	D	14.7	E	4.2	86.3	13.7

Note: Pediatrics included in all appropriate diagnoses.

Source: California Office of Statewide Health Planning and Development, 1988.

Table 3-7. Sample Community Hospital Cardiovascular Services Use Rate Projections: CY 1986 (actual), 1988, and 1993 (projected)

Product Line	Actual						Projected						CY 19xy (Projected)					
	Treated in Area		Out-Migration		Total		Treated in Area		Out-Migration		Total		Treated in Area		Out-Migration		Total	
	Discharge	Use Rate	Discharge	Frequency	Discharge	Incidence	Discharge	Use Rate	Discharge	Frequency	Discharge	Incidence	Discharge	Use Rate	Discharge	Frequency	Discharge	Incidence
Medical	2,575	17.11	291	1.93	2,866	19.04	2,851	17.17	322	1.94	3,173	19.11	3,467	17.17	392	1.94	3,859	19.11
Surgical	503	3.34	159	1.06	662	4.40	557	3.35	176	1.06	733	4.41	677	3.35	214	1.06	891	4.41
Total	3,078	20.45	450	2.99	3,528	23.44	3,407	20.52	498	3.00	3,906	23.52	4,145	20.52	606	3.00	4,751	23.52

Notes:
Total 1986 population = 150,489
Total 1988 population = 166,598
Total 1993 population = 202,646
Use rates = discharges per 1,000 population.
Assumes no changes in out-migration frequency 1988 to 1993.
Service/market area equals nine–zip code area.

Sources: California Office of State Health Planning and Development (OSHPD); National Planning Data Corp.

Inpatient and Outpatient Data

The tremendous growth of the outpatient market is influencing all areas of health care, including cardiovascular services. Although inpatient cardiac services continue to dominate the market, outpatient technologies — cardiac catheterization, echocardiography, nuclear cardiography, cardiac MRI, and conventional stress testing and EKGs — pose a threat to that dominance. All of these services are now offered in physicians' offices.

Because these outpatient procedures are not uniformly reported in as detailed a fashion as hospital discharges, accurate outpatient data are virtually nonexistent, and this situation seriously limits market analysis. Nevertheless, it is important to develop local or state use rates or use rate assumptions, which may be available from governmental agencies. For example, many states monitor utilization and compliance of outpatient services and require reporting of these statistics from individual hospitals. These reports can be analyzed to determine the number of procedures performed in a state or in a particular region. When compared with population data available for the study region, these utilization figures help in estimating regional outpatient use rates.

New technology may also contribute to the lack of data. This is due to the unfortunate time lapse between adoption of new technology and availability of statistical reports on its utilization. For example, several years passed before PTCA was reported separately from cardiac catheterization.

Usage Rates

Usage rates for cardiovascular services commonly are analyzed per 1,000 population. For example, when a usage rate for open-heart surgery is quoted as 1 per 1,000 per year, of every 1,000 persons in a given population, one underwent open-heart surgery during the 12-month period being studied.

Note that use rates differ from incidence rates in a given population because *use rates* refer only to procedures performed within the market area; use rates ignore patient origin. For example, a large urban area with regional treatment facilities may have a higher use rate because patients from surrounding rural communities may travel to the facilities in the urban center to receive services, either by choice or by necessity.

To measure the impact of this in-migration, the region for which use rates are being calculated should be as large as possible. A larger geographic area generally will encompass larger and smaller communities and programs, thereby minimizing the distortion resulting from patient migration and the loss of the related frequency data. These rates should then be compared to statewide or regional rates to test the reasonableness of the data and to identify significant differences in data.

In the absence of adequate local, regional, or state use rates, a volume of 4.0 diagnostic catheterizations per 1,000, 1.0 cardiac surgeries per 1,000, and 1.0 PTCAs per 1,000 may be used. These are conservative annual rates, substantiated in many mature markets (see discussion in chapter 2 and utilization rates in tables 1-6 and 1-8).

Analyzing usage rates can be difficult; for example, they frequently vary, and there is no objective way to determine whether the variation is significant or easily explainable. If a usage rate in a rural area is lower than in an urban area, for example, one of at least four factors could explain the difference: The rural population is not adequately served by this service, the rural population is healthier, the urban area rate is inflated due to in-migration from rural areas, or some combination of the three factors. Because it is difficult and sometimes impossible to separate objective and subjective reasons for use rate variations, it is important that the analysis seeks to explain variations rationally.

Once use rates have been combined with population figures for the service area, the market for CV services can be quantified and projections made for the growth of the market over a time period on the basis of population changes.

Current Referral Volume

To evaluate future demand for a cardiac catheterization laboratory, hospitals should begin by tracking patients presently transferred to other hospitals for cardiac catheterization. Referring cardiologists who intend to support the program often are willing to document their procedure volume and estimate the volume of cases they would have performed in the catheterization laboratory had one been available. Similarly, referring primary care physicians generally are willing to document or estimate their volume of patients referred for catheterization and verify where those patients were referred.

If a hospital already has a cardiac catheterization laboratory but is considering the addition of a cardiac surgery program, participating cardiologists should be asked to document the number or percentage of catheterization cases referred to, or performed at, a full-service cardiovascular program; the number or percentage of interventional cardiology cases referred to, or performed at, a full-service program by type of procedure; and the number or percentage of cardiac surgeries performed on their patients, again by procedure. It may be helpful to generate data on the hospital where each procedure was performed and on the physician involved in each case. This will help assess possible impact on competitors, which in turn will help gauge their competitive response to a new program.

Like virtually all other predominantly outpatient diagnostic procedures, noninvasive cardiology procedures are difficult if not impossible to quantify. This is true despite progress being made in identifying the frequency of all outpatient services. This difficulty is tied to several causes.

First of all, noninvasive cardiology procedures are split between inpatient and outpatient delivery points. Hospitals routinely document inpatient services but may not detail adequately information on outpatient services. Second, noninvasive cardiology procedures are performed in the offices of cardiologists, who generally do not report their procedure volume. Third, the incidence of use for various noninvasive procedures seems to vary considerably with location; and the literature suggests that, as in other procedures, physicians control the use of these procedures.

It can be expected that echocardiography and nuclear cardiography, the more expensive noninvasive procedure modalities, increasingly will become the focus of new development. Therefore, hospitals should facilitate all attempts to gather use information for these important procedures in order to gain a competitive advantage. As medical claims data become computerized and these data files are merged for analysis, virtually all procedures (regardless of cost, importance, or service location) will be quantified.

Competitors

All health care providers, regardless of their mission, size, or ownership, must contend with actual or potential competition as a consequence of factors such as oversupply or undersupply of resources, horizontal integration (such as a hospital purchasing another hospital) and vertical integration (such as a hospital purchasing a home care agency), and so forth.

Competition has transformed strategy formulation, strategic planning, and marketing from theoretical concepts into mandatory behaviors. Put another way, competition is one environmental variable that drives hospital strategy, which in turn drives an organization's operational and marketing activities. Strategy and ongoing operations will reflect other considerations to be sure, but the role of competition as a variable will always be significant and will increase in direct relation to its impact on the hospital.

The prevailing concepts of competition are derived from economics and involve the rivalry among independent entities in pursuit of the same objective—or a struggle of two or more contenders for marketplace dominance. However, competition among health care organizations cannot be characterized so simply. Although in many respects a mature industry, in terms of classic economic theory, health care behaves as an "emerging business," characterized by technological innovations, shifts in relative cost relationships, emergence of new consumer needs, and other socioeconomic changes.

The bottom-line characteristic of an emerging industry is that there are no rules of the game. Therefore, competition becomes difficult to identify, assess, and, ultimately, use as the basis of strategy formulation. Nevertheless, because competitor analysis is critical in assessing a new program or service, the following questions must be addressed:

- Who are the hospital's direct, indirect, and future competitors?
- What market position strategies are used by competitors?
- What are the competitors' key characteristics?
- What are the strengths and weaknesses of each competitor?
- How is each competitor likely to respond to a strategic action?
- What other forces affect competition?

Direct, Indirect, and Future Competitors

Generally, competition is understood in the context of hospital versus hospital, but physicians, specifically cardiologists and primary care physicians, are also important competitors as well as influencers of other competitors. Only cardiovascular surgery must take place within a hospital; all other services are — or will be — available on an outpatient basis, which means they can be performed in physicians' offices. Echocardiography is perhaps the best historical example of a service in which cardiologists have been potent competitors to hospitals. Because echocardiography is a relatively inexpensive technology, cardiologists and physician groups have been quick to invest in equipment once their volume reaches the break-even point. Furthermore, ultrasonography has become a profitable component of the typical cardiologist's practice, leaving hospital programs with the inpatient market and services to low-pay or no-pay patients. Certainly, other diagnostic tests are dominated by physicians, and cardiac catheterization may soon follow in many market areas.

Recognizing that historical competitors will not retain their position of dominance is helpful in the process of identifying competitors. For example, medical groups, HMOs, even large employers may become competitive factors in the future health care environment. Assessing the competitive environment is not an isolated task but an ongoing process of competitor surveillance.

Market Position Strategies Used by Competitors

Positioning is a marketing concept of manipulating a program's image within the mind of the target audience, without changing the service.

An effort must be made to understand fully the positioning strategy used by each competitor. The hospital that positions itself as "the low-cost leader," "the high-quality program," "the high-volume program," or "the physician-friendly provider" should do so only after examining the positioning strategies of competitors in the market. This is particularly important if two market competitors are vying for the same position.

Competitors' Key Characteristics

What are the competitors' service mix, utilization, market share, financial position, facilities, technology, and medical staff composition?

These are some of the competitor data that can be gathered over time. Typically, this information is of general interest but provides an important outline for understanding the competitor. Monitoring changes in these parameters can also help signal an imminent change in overall direction. For example, if a competitor that historically has been technologically lax begins to enhance its services and facilities, it may be attempting to build a foundation to recruit a new physician or physician group.

Similar competitor profiles should be maintained on physicians, particularly those who compete with physicians loyal to the planning hospital. Toward this end, the following elements can be monitored: patient volumes; admitting trends; contractual arrangements with hospitals for emergency room call and interpretations; their office technologies, unique services, or capabilities; partner affiliations; patient services contracts; and so on. These components are used to examine competitors among members of the medical community.

Competitors' Strengths and Weaknesses

Cataloging the strengths and weaknesses of hospital and physician competitors is perhaps the most important task in comprehending the competitive environment. An admittedly subjective process, this analysis will promote an understanding of a hospital's own opportunities and vulnerabilities, which when combined with an appreciation of its strengths and weaknesses will ultimately lead to a prescription for strategic action. In many respects this ongoing "sizing up" of the competition is at the heart of the strategic and competitive process.

Competitors' Response to Strategic Action

For every strategic action, there is a reaction in the market; often that reaction is from competitors. Although a competitor's response may not be equal and opposite, it will be forthcoming for every action taken. Anticipating that response is an often-overlooked step in the analysis, a step that despite the difficulty attached is a worthwhile task. For example, adding a catheterization laboratory makes good sense in a market where cardiologists complain about scheduling difficulties with existing laboratories, but the likelihood that someone else will add a catheterization laboratory must also be taken into account.

Calculating competitor actions must occur not only in response to others' actions (*defensive* strategic actions) but also in response to market opportunity (*offensive* strategic actions). Both actions influence the assessment of the market and the formulation of strategy. If, for example, one hospital identifies an opportunity to enter the catheterization market by setting up a catheterization laboratory, a competitor with an existing catheterization program may add a laboratory in response to this perceived threat, thereby significantly changing the strategic environment. Such a scenario will require the prospective new entrant to secure firm support from catheterization cardiologists.

Other Forces That Affect Competition

To facilitate identification and analysis of competitors and to address the issues outlined above, managers must examine the multitude of forces that drive competition and hence hospital strategy and planning. Remember, successful planning is always market-driven, meaning that the realities of the local marketplace dictate strategy. In a competitive environment, multiple, overlapping forces are at work; these forces, which affect strategy, are outlined in figure 3-2 and detailed below.

Figure 3-2. Forces That Affect Competition and Strategy

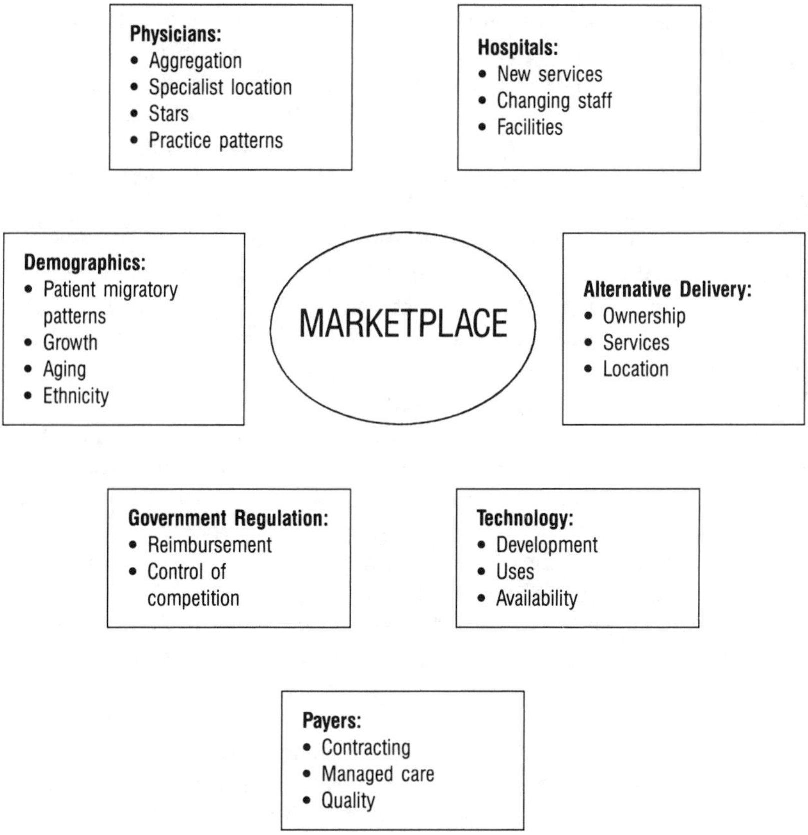

Hospitals
Obviously, the first place to look for organized competition is other hospitals within and surrounding the targeted service area. These hospitals should initially be profiled in terms of facilities and services including, of course, CV services such as noninvasive cardiology testing services and their ownership, cardiac catheterization, cardiac surgery, cardiac rehabilitation, and so forth. This leads to identifying service gaps that can be exploited, such as lack of a catheterization laboratory in a key market area or the opportunity to add open-heart surgery.

An effort should be made to gather as much initial information as possible from formal and informal sources, including members of the hospital's medical staff and other sources in the local community.

Competitor profiles should include a listing of cardiovascular facilities, including cardiac rehabilitation units; number and type of catheterization laboratories; specific catheterization laboratory services available, such as digital subtraction angiography and electrophysiology; and any plans for the addition of cardiovascular equipment, including equipment for the catheterization laboratory and noninvasive cardiology. Cardiovascular surgery facilities also must be identified as well as CSICU space, telemetry (monitored) beds, and so on. Also, the facility's participation in ventures with other physicians such as mobile catheterization laboratories and cardiac diagnostic imaging centers should be examined. This information is helpful not only in gauging gaps but also in forecasting competitors' future activities.

To the extent possible, a definitive list should be compiled of cardiologists and cardiology groups supporting the competitor's program; a description of each cardiologist's primary care referral base and details on the political and organizational structures at the hospitals, including medical directorships, heart institute structures, and the like. In urban markets, similar information, although difficult to obtain, should be gathered on cardiac surgeons. Because physicians control the flow of patients, the more that is known about how the referral network functions, the more effective the strategy will be to modify it. This information must be gathered regularly over time, and preferably from the physicians themselves.

Volume indicators for the catheterization laboratory and surgery program, as well as other pertinent information, should be monitored in detail as regularly as possible. All these data should be compiled and updated at least annually so that the competitor profile remains current. A system should be established and responsibility assigned to ensure the smooth flow of this ongoing process.

Special attention should be given to anticipating new services, changes within the medical community, and new facilities and technology planned by competing hospitals. Although the competitor's historic position is important, its evolving role is even more important.

Physicians
As already noted, more and more physicians are competing with hospitals. It is also clear that whereas physicians and physician groups can be allies, they also can become competitors, particularly with respect to the development of new facilities and services, and with respect to other physicians who remain loyal to the planning hospital's current program. Therefore, understanding the political issues that affect the medical community is another key to successful strategy formulation.

The trend toward physician aggregation, or grouping together, for a common goal is evident at varying levels across the country. Because of the consolidation of economic and political power, the tendency for physicians to aggregate into single-specialty and multispecialty medical groups stimulates further competition between hospitals and physicians. At the same time, it increases the potential for strategic cooperation for mutual benefit. In any case, the aggregation of physicians and the migration of physicians within and between groups — as well as the consequent relationship changes from a referral perspective — are important considerations in planning a new service or expanding an existing one.

Examining the relationship of specialists within the larger physician community is also important for planning purposes. For example, the traditional relationship between primary care physicians — who refer patients — and cardiology specialists is an obvious factor to study.

Physician practice patterns are another emerging force. In an era when hospitals will compete for cardiovascular business increasingly on the basis of quality and cost, the practice patterns of physicians who provide care within the program directly affect that program's ability to compete. Therefore, if hospitals hope to compete successfully for managed care contracts, it is essential that they be prepared to develop aggressive and politically acceptable methods to exclude from contracting those physicians who consistently fail to deliver high-quality and cost-effective patient care.

Finally, "star" or "magnet" physicians can have a tremendous impact on the ability of specific hospitals to compete. Star physicians stand out on the basis of their abilities to deliver high-quality clinical care and to manage relationships successfully. *Some star physicians have made their mark within a marketplace not because they have superior clinical skills, but because they have good clinical skills and world-class referral and management skills.*

Differences in physicians' clinical skills will diminish in importance as cardiac specialty services become more commonplace. The physician who can manage relationships with referral groups will become more marketable and more valuable strategically.

Strategies that block — but do not prevent — physicians and medical groups from entering the invasive cardiology market must be acted on aggressively. *Blocking* implies creating disincentives for the physicians to enter these markets and incentives for them to work with the planning hospital. For the hospital, then, these blocking mechanisms include entering the market first, offering joint venture opportunities, contracting aggressively for patient services, and so forth. To be successful, not only must these strategies be legal and ethical, they must meet the needs of the physicians. Physician involvement in developing these strategies, therefore, is essential.

Alternative Delivery
As already mentioned, a variety of alternative delivery systems can positively or negatively impact the cardiovascular program and competitors. The most important developments to observe will be the growth of mobile cardiac catheterization laboratories and the formation of freestanding cardiac catheterization laboratories in cardiologists' offices. Three trends are promoting these developments: the dissemination of cardiologists into more remote sites, the aggregation of cardiologists into larger groups with increased economic clout and capability, and the declining income from professional cardiac services as a result of competition and shrinking reimbursement levels.

Should cardiac catheterization go the way of echocardiography, the market for hospital-operated catheterization facilities will focus on inpatient services and on treatment of the underinsured. This declining volume and the shifting of more profitable patients into physician laboratories will place economic pressure on current programs. At present, nothing legally or ethically prevents this from occurring; therefore, hospitals will be challenged to develop proactive strategies to minimize the negative impact of this trend.

Mobile and freestanding catheterization laboratories can be developed by hospitals without joint venturing. Strategies should be examined that enhance availability and improve scheduling for cardiologists near these facilities. Consideration should also be given to bundling other cardiovascular diagnostic services and cardiac rehabilitation with these services, including the development of mobile noninvasive diagnostic services. Finally, partnerships with hospitals that do not have the most up-to-date cardiovascular services should also be reevaluated.

Technology
The effect of new technology on data availability, noninvasive service gaps, and hospital–physician competition already has been cited. New technology exerts other influences on the competitive environment. For example, adding a positron emission tomography (PET) center or entering the atherectomy business early in the product life cycle can influence a facility's referral patterns. Although the investment is significant and the payoff questionable for major technology initiatives, the technological horizon still must be routinely and vigorously scanned for technologies that may compete with current services or produce an opportunity for the current program.

Demographics

Described elsewhere in this chapter, demographics need only be recapped here. As the foundation for the planning process they directly affect conclusions drawn about the potential need and utilization of cardiovascular services. Understanding demographic trends in terms of growth, age and sex cohorts, race, and location of the population is important, as is anticipating patient migratory patterns.

Government Regulation

Governmental regulatory agencies can profoundly affect competition. Certificate-of-need (CON) legislation must be a consideration; for example, changes must be anticipated in those states where CON legislation is undergoing review. If CON is waning, the impact for hospitals with existing CV services (particularly the potential influx of new entrants into the market) must be assessed. In those states considering tightening CON regulations in general or specifically as they apply to cardiovascular services, different competition realities must be anticipated. Specific regulations concerning cardiovascular services (for example, minimum volume requirements to retain licensure) are not unlikely; ongoing attention will be paid to program volume until the focus shifts to program outcome regardless of volume. It is reasonable to anticipate at least some discussion of these targeted regulatory efforts.

The potential for Medicare-sponsored regionalization of cardiovascular surgery is an obvious example of how the regulatory environment can significantly impact the competitive environment.

Payers

The impact of managed care on a competitive environment for cardiovascular services is increasing at a remarkable rate. As mentioned in chapter 1, this impact will stem from insurers, employers, and managed care firms such as utilization review firms and TPAs. Managed care can be expected to be a major force in the distribution of cardiovascular services in the future.

The principal effect of managed care will be a stabilization of prices, eliminating major price differences between high-cost and low-cost providers in a particular market. Price stabilization will make cost-based competition increasingly difficult, which will become particularly apparent when the comparatively low impact of fixed costs on cardiovascular surgery is considered. Fixed costs such as facilities, plant, and equipment are an important financial consideration, but not significant enough to eliminate the smaller program from the typical CV market.

Specialty managed care or specialty preferred provider organizations (SPPOs) will emerge as a dominant force. Even though other product lines will become the subject of SPPOs, cardiovascular services likely will be first because they command the largest share of a health insurer's expenditures and are the easiest to package. This is so because the bulk of those services are accounted for in seven relatively homogeneous DRGs: DRG 104, valve procedure with catheterization; DRG 105, valve procedure without cath; DRG 106 coronary bypass with catheterization; DRG 107, coronary bypass without catheterization; DRG 112, including PTCA; DRGs 124 and 125, inpatient cardiac catheterization.

An effort will be made to minimize the number of SPPO participants so as to increase the volume of patients channeled to each, thereby increasing the attractiveness of the contract.

Summary

Local market assessment serves as a foundation in planning a cardiovascular program — whether new, expanded, or revised services. Four stages are involved in the process: prestudy, data collection and analysis, determination of findings, and developing conclusions and recommendations.

In considering external forces — factors outside the hospital environment — an assessment needs to look closely at several areas of market influence. These include (but are not limited to):

- Defining the geographic boundaries served
- Analyzing that area's demographics — population, age, racial makeup, sex
- Determining market share — what actual of potential percentage of total market area can be captured
- Studying inpatient and outpatient data (more difficult to attain but can be analyzed from government reports)
- Projecting usage rates (must not be confused with incidence rates), taking into consideration patient migration patterns
- Tracking patient referral volume — both for the host hospital and other hospitals in the area
- Analyzing competitors — who they are, what services they provide, with what technology, medical staff composition, strengths and weaknesses, and such

Performing an accurate, effective assessment of the local market relies on accurate information. Where facts are not easily obtained, anecdotal information — patient and/or staff surveys, hospital medical records, for example — must be prepared. Failure to gather and assess data *at the beginning* will virtually doom a cardiovascular program.

Chapter 4

Program Strategy Development

Once the market has been assessed, program opportunities determined, and goals set, the hospital planning team is ready to develop a program strategy. In the past, hospital leadership planned and developed programs by designing mission statements and strategies that applied to the *entire* hospital. However, planning at the *program* level—that is, planning strategy that is tailored for a particular clinical service—is becoming more commonplace. This is a direct result of recognition that individual hospital units (or modules) can make plans on the basis of the forces at play in their respective markets. Viewed from a different perspective, successful hospitals are focusing their growth and advancement on the development of thriving specialty service lines, such as cardiovascular services.

Although a number of methods can be used to develop strategy for restructuring or implementing CV services, this chapter presents one, which uses the strategic action matrix, that shows how it is used to identify the principal prerequisites for achieving desired outcomes. The model program presented later in the chapter will help planners design a program as well as identify opportunities for program development or gaps in competitors' strengths and weaknesses.

To design a successful CV program development strategy, the planning team must include a mechanism for regular plan updating. To do so, a framework for decision making is needed to move the facility steadily toward its stated goals; this framework is provided by a concise vision (mission) statement. The most effective mission statements incorporate specific and attainable goals and full commitment to the vision.

This chapter covers six major topics:

1. Strategy formulation (includes development of a market-based mission statement and a product line inventory; also cites barriers to strategy)

2. Strategic action matrix (policy statement, moving from concept to action and tactics)
3. Gateways to successful implementation (selecting and prioritizing actions)
4. Development and implementation (role of leadership and teamwork)
5. Model CV program
6. Elements of a successful strategy program

Strategy Formulation

Warren Bennis has identified several functions of a leader, the most important of which is to create and communicate a vision for the organization.[1] It is difficult enough to *formulate* an appropriate vision but even more difficult to *communicate* it to the rest of the organization. If not communicated, such vision will fail to galvanize the organization into action.

Values emerge as a direct result of the vision. These values in turn affect the establishment of *convictions*. Together, values and convictions permeate the organization and provide the framework for setting objectives. This unity allows for programwide decision making based on objectives that move the organization steadily toward its goals. Homogeneity also provides an atmosphere of synergy throughout the organization, in that everyone works toward a common goal; they have a say in the process and a stake in the outcome.

The end products of this *value chain* (the relationship between vision, value systems, convictions, and objectives) are the organizational objectives (see figure 4-1). Objectives are the essential foundation for effective decision making.

The following is an example of a vision statement, with specific objectives for a cardiovascular program:

> The Good Guy Heart Center will be the largest cardiovascular program in Hillsboro by the end of 1994. By then volume will have reached 850 cardiovascular surgeries, 2,500 diagnostic catheterizations, and 900 angioplasties. We will have an integrated, state-of-the-art program while staying within the capital budget. This will occur through prudent selection of technologies to develop. Our services will be of the highest documentable quality and our case costs will be below $25,000 for surgery and below $7,000 for PTCA. Our outpatient catheterization rate will be 55 percent. By the end of next year we will have in place 15 additional patient services contracts, contracted at rates that produce demonstrated profits.

This statement is simple, understandable, and easily communicated. Although vision statements are often thought of as being lofty and ambiguous, in reality

Figure 4-1. The Value Chain

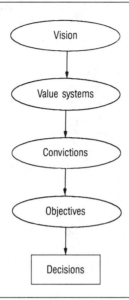

they must be realistic and precise to serve as valuable planning tools. Most important, they must be communicated, understood, and agreed to by a significant percentage of the staff. This conforms with a principle of strategy formation: *strategy must always be simple without being simplistic.* This modest statement, difficult to carry off in practice, makes the continuous focus on strategy an imperative for the successful management team.

The process of formulating strategy varies with time and place. As concluded from chapter 3, strategy always must evolve from the current market. Although certain innovations in management and technology that are separate from the market (the concept of product line management popular in the 1980s or advancements in echocardiography developed in the early 1990s) may seem to have direct application, initiation *into* the market must always be environmentally based, that is, market-driven. Strategy for cardiovascular services often must rest on the more mundane and parochial aspects of environment, such as local politics or regional competition.

The strategy formulation process grows out of, and overlaps with, the four stages of market assessment described in chapter 3. Once stage 1 (prestudy) and stage 2 (data collection and analysis) are completed, the next two phases (determination of findings and development of conclusions and recommendations, respectively) merge with strategic planning, which culminates in what is, in effect, stage 5 — implementation. The four stages then can be summarized in four reports, correspondingly titled as follows:

1. *Findings:* A summary report of the findings of a market assessment might include an external and an internal environmental assessment; for the most part, findings will be objective statements of facts uncovered in quantitative research but may include summaries of subjective factors uncovered in interviews or other qualitative research.
2. *Conclusions:* This analytical report should identify principal barriers to successful formation and implementation of strategy as well as statements of policies and principles underlying the program.
3. *Recommendations:* This report elaborates extensively on the strategies and tactics required to implement the principles and policies established in the conclusions stage; recommendations may be more subjective than findings or conclusions but must be tied to, and emerge from, conclusions drawn from those findings.
4. *Implementation plan:* This report defines how recommended strategies and tactics will be implemented (by whom, by what date, with what resources, for what expected outcomes); the plan should detail evaluation mechanisms to monitor implementation and define feedback loops for ongoing adjustments in the original plans.

Advancing through these stages ensures that strategy will be market-based. The market (including internal and external circumstances) is the fundamental ingredient of the situation audit, described later in this chapter.

Figure 4-2 illustrates this four-stage strategy formulation/reporting process for a representative CV program. The balance of this chapter will examine the activities involved at each stage. *Findings* involve analyzing structural variables, organizational elements, product line inventory, and market information. Structural variables are discussed later in the chapter as they are delineated in a model CV program, followed by an examination of organizational elements. Product line inventory and marketing information are discussed briefly here. *Conclusions* encompasses barriers to strategy formulation and a strategic action matrix for developing statements of policy, strategy, and tactics. *Recommendations* emerge as gateways to strategy implementation and, finally, to *plan implementation.*

Product Line Inventory

The *product line inventory* is a tool to assess program elements that are in place and identify elements that may need to be added. Because cardiovascular programs are entirely full service, it is appropriate to examine candidate products, such as catheterization laboratories, for their strengths, weaknesses, and applicability for program inclusion. Given the resources available within the hospital or within the market, it will not be feasible to provide every product. For example, certain procedures require specially trained physicians, whereas others, such as transplants, require particularly large market areas.

Used as a tool for scheduling and prioritizing opportunities based on defined variables (for example, market served, facilities needed, or staffing allocation), the product line inventory serves to educate planners about possible program development within the market. It also can help document that the hospital has a relatively sophisticated program in place. Product line inventory is discussed further in chapter 5.

Market Information

As discussed in chapter 3, findings are derived by analyzing the market for data (market size, market share, migration, competition). The more data that can be digested, the more complete the analysis will be and, therefore, the more concise the objectives and action plans.

Figure 4-2. Strategy Formulation Process

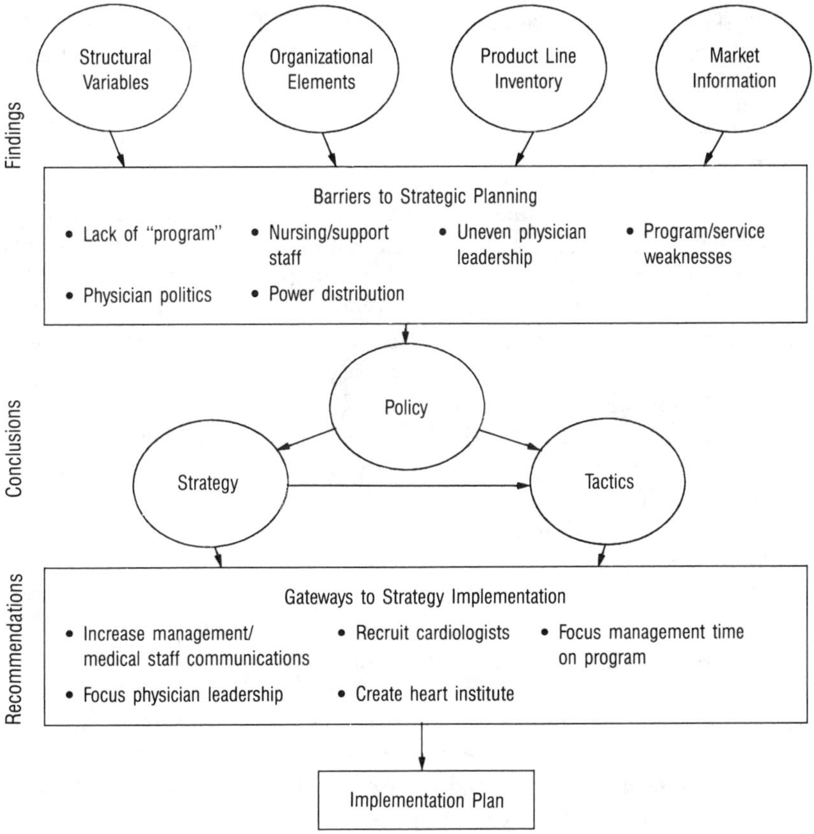

Barriers to Strategy Formulation

Because strategy must be simple, it is imperative that efforts be focused and that issues be prioritized. Reviewing the environment invariably will lead to identifying certain inhibiting factors, or barriers, that can jeopardize program strategy. A plan that takes account of barriers also will prompt hospital executives to confer enabling authority where needed to maintain momentum and overcome inertia. Some barriers are listed in figure 4-2.

Strategic Action Matrix

The *strategic action matrix* combines the highest level of broad vision statements with the strategies and tactics proposed for implementing them (figure 4-3, p. 88). The vision statement is broken down into individual *policy statements,* which derive from guiding principles. *Strategies* are crafted for each policy statement, and a number of *tactics* are outlined for each strategy. Thus the matrix links ideas regarding future directions and accomplishments with the actions needed to realize them.

Policy Statements

Before attempting to formulate an overall mission or vision statement for the cardiovascular program, such as the one quoted at the outset of this chapter, an effort should be made to get key stakeholders to agree on an outline of the principles to be digested, synthesized, and summarized in the vision statement. Formulating policy statements from guiding principles will in turn drive formulation of related strategies and tactics.

The formulation of policy statements begins by reviewing the findings of the market assessment, filtering out trivial market data, and concentrating on the factors that will make a difference in forging strategy. Incidental market data should be attached as a report addendum.

Market analysis from an objective and a subjective standpoint can be summarized around specific strategy propositions: strengths, weaknesses, opportunities, and threats — *SWOT analysis* (based on Steiner's now-famous *WOTS-UP analysis* of weaknesses, opportunities, threats, and strengths underlying planning). Steiner is also credited with the concept of the *situation audit,* which refers to assessment of the environment including the internal and external environments.[2] The internal audit produces an array of strengths and weaknesses, whereas the external analysis generates awareness of opportunities and threats found in the external environment (marketplace). The examination of SWOTs can be displayed in a variety of formats, including that found in figure 4-4 (p. 90).

As a tool, SWOT analysis is simple, widely used, and extremely beneficial. Furthermore, it lends itself well to group processes whereby members of the team are asked to identify and later discuss and/or prioritize strengths, weaknesses, opportunities, and threats. This technique also provides a forum for discussing the major issues that must be agreed on prior to formation of the vision statement. Examples of the sorts of guiding principles that could emerge from this process are shown in figure 4-5 (p. 91).

Policy statements elaborate on the guiding principles and are not one-for-one translations of each specific principle; nevertheless, when fully implemented the policies are supportive of the principles and will realize their fulfillment. Thus policy statements are the first entry in the sample strategic action matrix in figure 4-3.

Strategies

The strategic action matrix is designed to identify concepts that become increasingly activity oriented as they flow from left to right on the matrix. Note that each policy statement (guide to strategic thinking) is followed by several strategies. The strategies, although more action oriented than the policy statement, are not specific in the activity or steps required; nor are they necessarily quantifiable.

Tactics

Each strategy is implemented by launching a series of tactics. Depending on the level of analysis, these tactics will be action oriented and can be specific and time targeted. This section of the strategic action matrix can serve as the vehicle for development of management objectives and action plans that can be used as the basis on which managers will be held accountable for implementing their assigned tasks.

Gateways to Strategy Implementation

It is not uncommon for a strategic action matrix to yield literally hundreds of concepts and activities. But because they all cannot be communicated or tracked adequately and because it is unlikely they all will be accomplished, only the *critical issues and actions* required for a cardiovascular program must be identified. These critical success factors will be the gateways to successful strategy and, ultimately, a successful program. Although many issues may be important, the number of gateways should be restricted to a maximum of six or eight (samples are shown in figure 4-2).

Figure 4-3. Cardiovascular Services: Strategic Action Matrix

Policy Statements	Strategies	Tactics
1. Case volume targets will be established and communicated for cardiovascular surgery, interventional cardiology, and diagnostic strategies	A. Set targets at 450 surgeries, 500 PTCAs, and 1,800 diagnostic caths	(1) Estimate referral capacities (2) Assess hospital patient origins (3) Target key markets (4) Initially set medical staff politics aside (5) Develop complex PTCA privilege plan (6) Create ER "leakage" prevention plan
	B. Adjust targets with input from cardiologists	(1) Secure physician commitment to volume targets (2) Develop hospital–physician joint marketing
2. A concerted effort will be made to measure and improve quality in cardiovascular surgery and cardiology	A. Develop conventions for measuring the quality of cardiology and cardiovascular surgery based on nationally accepted protocols	(1) Cardiologists to define quality with input from surgeon, anesthesia, and clinical staff, and vice versa (2) Criteria communicated to medical staff committee structure (3) Results and actions properly communicated
	B. Establish mechanisms to improve and document quality	(1) Develop educational options for staff cardiologists (2) Enhance non-CV hospital-based physician support (e.g., pulmonary, infectious disease, nephrology) (3) Increase cardiologists' postoperative involvement (4) Examine recruitment alternatives (5) Initiate corrective measures as required (6) Communicate results as appropriate (7) Ensure in-house availability

3. Case costs for all major cardiovascular DRGs will be reduced to competitive levels while maintaining profitability	A. Create substantial and understandable data base	(1) Examine existing information system reports (2) Identify key cardiovascular DRGs (3) Review external competitive information
	B. Assess case charges	(1) Break down by DRG (2) Categorize charges by department or responsibility center (3) Evaluate outliers (4) Compare historically
	C. Set case targets	(1) Review contracting environment (2) Compare hospital charges (3) Compare state charges
	D. Evaluate case costs	(1) Prepare cost model

Figure 4-4. Scenario One: SWOT Analysis and Critical Success Factors (Regional Perspective)

Internal		External	
Strengths	**Weaknesses**	**Opportunities**	**Threats**
• Physical presence is tangible • Meets the market vision of an institute • Provides tangible evidence of performance • Focused management • Data become information • Promotion is targeted and reflects program substance • Improved quality • Lower cost/better price • Improved margin	• Expensive • Disruptive to organization reporting structures • Budgeting not consistent with current budgeting process • Space availability • Clinical research (high profile)	• Develop relationship with primary care physicians (PCPs) and referral cardiologists • Develop relationships with payers • Focus on measurement and documentation of quality • Educate payers, referring physicians, and public on the issues they should decide • Responsive to sensitive issues and PCP's feeling about treatment	• Perceived focus on cardiovascular services upsetting to other product lines • Competitor response

Critical Success Factors

• Hospital CEOs to focus on other lines
• Separate entity from either hospital
• VP-level manager reports directly to board and focuses full-time on institute success
• Executive medical advisory board chaired by medical director and includes representatives from each hospital's program along with PCPs
• Develop outreach program to focus public education in PCPs' offices
• VP manages relationships around physicians and clinical departments
• Clinical departments report to hospital service line managers, who report to VP of heart institute
• Standard treatment protocol (STP) reduces cost and improves quality
• STP process is monitored and managed on an ongoing basis
• Data support available
• Develop patient relations program (handbook, patient rep, follow-up, and data base)

Figure 4-5. Cardiovascular Services: Sample Guiding Principles

1. The cardiovascular program is essential to the success of General Medical Center.

2. General Medical Center will be the leading provider of cardiovascular services. This will require a program that supports 450 cardiac surgeries, 500 PTCAs, and 1,800 diagnostic catheterizations.

3. Strong and competent leadership, both physicians and administrators, is essential and therefore will be fostered and facilitated.

4. An organization will emerge that will allow cardiac services to function as a *program:* articulating objectives, crafting strategy, and implementing tactics.

5. Interventional cardiology will play a larger role in the cardiovascular program's success in the future.

6. Managed care will continue to be a major force in the cardiovascular market in the near future, and case costs and documented quality therefore will be key strategic variables.

7. Managing relationships with referring physicians, payers, patients, the community, and team members will be the principal ingredients for success in this market.

8. Success can be achieved only in an optimistic and enthusiastic environment.

9. Although turbulent political environments must be avoided to allow the focus and energy necessary to excel in a competitive market, risks will be taken.

10. Constant communication will be maintained among program stakeholders in order to engender trust, foster creativity, facilitate problem solving, build teams, remove barriers, reduce resistance, and allow a strong and calm center to emerge within the program.

Strategy Development and Implementation

Identifying creative strategy options and selecting appropriate directions for implementation are the product of knowledge, intuition, experience, and wisdom. Because all of these attributes are rarely embodied in one individual, strategy is developed most effectively through a group.

It is important that strategy be forged not simply as a vote "by majority rule" of program participants. As noted throughout this book in several contexts, successful implementation requires a leader and the regular application of leadership skills to guide the decisions necessary for crafting effective strategy.

Implementation is the test of a management team, for a less-than-optimal decision or strategy that is well implemented is far better than a brilliant strategy that is poorly implemented. Therefore, how the management team administers details and responds to market and environmental nuances once implementation is under way is a measure of team skill. Concepts of cardiovascular program implementation are discussed more fully in chapter 7.

A useful strategy is to compare the recommendations for the subject program with a model cardiovascular program to gauge similarities and differences between the two. If the model is based on a full-service program with numerous options, a thorough discussion of the structural variables of a model cardiovascular program will ensue.

Structural Variables of a Model Cardiovascular Program

The *structural variables* of a clinical program are those factors required to transform a *service* into a *program* (a coordinated grouping of services) that can be qualitatively differentiated from disparate services. The variables shown in figure 4-6 are discussed here in terms of a model cardiovascular program.

The concept of a model program is difficult in that it must be understood in the context of a particular situation and circumstance and is subject to continual refinement and change. For example, the cardiovascular model for a large university hospital program is fundamentally different from that of a small community referral program. Depending on the unique characteristics of a hospital and its market, each situation will require a reconsideration and revision of the elements in this format. The cardiovascular models in figures 4-6 (p. 94) and 4-7 (p. 96) are offered only as examples of how to use this analytical tool.

The model program methodology is beneficial in three ways. First, the discussion and debate necessary to arrive at an agreement on program elements and visualize the program from the perspective of the model can help participants evaluate their own program by previewing a number of variables. This results in agreement as to "what *our* program ideally should look like." Second, the self-analysis necessary to describe a program in terms of these elements can be a rewarding process in and of itself. Finally, this process can be applied to competitive programs at other hospitals, thus identifying gaps in the competition.

Structural variables for a model CV program (shown in figure 4-6) are detailed below.

Medical Staff Leadership

In the model program, leadership revolves around the medical staff. Archetypical programs historically were built around a dominant cardiovascular surgeon, but newer programs are often built around a strong cardiologist or cardiology group. If no dominant individual or group exists, physicians compete—on the basis of skill and stature—for the leadership position, always keeping the needs of the program in mind. Management is supportive, complements leadership within the medical community, and works to capitalize on the strengths of the physicians and remedy any weaknesses.

The medical staff is supportive of the program, not only within the specialties directly affected by the program, but also throughout the organized medical staff and community. *This relationship with the medical community is a focus of regular efforts by the cardiovascular medical and management leadership.*

Individual physicians limit their autonomy for the benefit of the program in order to present a united organization rather than an assortment of individuals and independent practices. Cardiologists already will have formed single-specialty groups and established cordial working relationships.

Coordination

Throughout the strategy development process, including implementation, group orientation should be evident, with the needs of the *program* uppermost at each step in the decision-making processes. Without demonstrating a "group think" mentality, team members should show a healthy appreciation for, and regular examination of, the dynamics of individual and group needs.

Market Scope

The model CV program has access to a market that can support a wide array of services within the program and accommodate a variety of physicians. The market should be large enough to support growth and development. There will also be an adequate supply of primary care physicians with the potential to refer cardiovascular patients. The program will enhance relationships with the primary care community by having the capacity to handle the screening and evaluation procedures they prescribe for their patients.

Services/Facilities

The market supports an appropriate array of services and facilities. Cardiovascular programs/services are conveniently located for patients as well as non–hospital-based cardiologists. Scheduling is arranged such that cardiologists are drawn to the facilities.

Integration

Regular efforts are made to integrate the needs of various stakeholders — cardiac surgeons, invasive and interventional cardiologists, noninvasive cardiologists, cardiac anesthesiologists, pulmonologists, neurologists, other hospital-based physicians, primary care physicians, infectious disease physicians, nurses, therapists, technologists, and hospital department managers.

The model program is flexible enough that major groups have input and there is room for a variety of opinions. However, decisions can still be made expeditiously when time is of the essence.

Politics

With the number of high-powered individuals involved in planning and managing a cardiovascular program, politics *will* be an issue. However, the

Figure 4-6. Cardiovascular Program Structural Variables Analysis (Based on Interview Results)

Structural Variables	Model Program	Our Hospital	Competitor Hospital
Medical staff leadership	• Strong, singular, or competed for on basis of competence and stature • Supportive • Limited self-determination • Cardiologists aggregated	• No program leadership • Cardiologists lack organization • Strong hospital-based noninvasive cardiologist • Dissension • Mistrust • Quality assurance in question	• No program leadership • Cardiologists lack organization • Complacent • Contentious • Highly skilled • Solo practice mentality • Self-determination
Coordination	• Program orientation • Administration/physician	• Fragmented, conflicting	• Fragmented • Practice orientation • Many directions
Market position	• Volume available • Physician based • Clear market leader	• Excellent position • Growth market • Strong competition • No clear market leader	• Excellent location • Stable market • Strong competition
Services/facilities	• Convenient for patients • Attractive to itinerant cardiologists	• Disjointed • No distinguishing factors	• Not convenient • No distinguishing factors
Integration	• Individual/group • Consensus forum	• None	• Limited
Politics	• Healthy • Program centered	• Strong politics, very personal • Growing medical staff unrest	• Practice-centered
Primary care	• Accessed through campus or network • Outreach a priority	• Adequate • Independent practice association in place • Limited primary physician network	• Limited • Independent practice association in place • No strong plans for development
Identity	• Physician/group focused • Collaborative	• None	• None

Decision making	• Benevolent dictator or consensus driven • Based on program needs	• Fragmented • Change process unclear	• Fragmented and labored
Quality	• Principal strength • Internal • Collegial	• Good CV surgery mortality statistics • No quality assurance • Uncertain PTCA results	• Good CVS mortality statistics • Inconsistent cardiology quality
Managed care	• Anticipatory posture • A target	• Managed care is not a major force in this market • Lacks informal network	• Unclear strategy
Cost orientation/ management	• Increasingly cost oriented • Organized to facilitate	• High cost (case charge) • Poorly organized to respond	
Growth	• Ongoing focus • Competence driven	• No clear direction	• Not presently organized to respond • No clear direction or commitment to growth • Losing market share
Technology	• Appropriately prioritized • Individual physician driven	• State-of-the-art cardiology • Questionable CV surgery methods	• State-of-the-art cardiology • No CVS advantage
Marketing	• Network oriented • Nonpromotional • Directed at physicians	• Excellent promotion • Poor patient relations • Poor referring physician relations	• Poor promotion; response-oriented • Good patient relations • No strategy for referring physician development
Organization	• Program is present • Administrative/medical staff function for benefit of program	• Fragmented	• Fragmented

Figure 4-7. Cardiovascular Program Organizational Elements (Based on Interview Results)

	Organizational Elements of a Model Program	Our Hospital	Competitor Hospital
Cardiology	• Multiple • Group present • No primary care • On-site availability • Aggressive	• No group; many cardiologists • No primary care • In-house access • Limited responsibility • Uneven physician quality	• No group • No "loyal" dedicated invasive cardiologists • Quality is questioned by some • No on-site, hospital-affiliated invasive cardiology
Cardiovascular surgery	• Single group • Relationship oriented • Staff support • Accessible • Dedicated supervisor and coordinators • Dedicated space	• Multiple groups • Limited relationship management • Staff support • Accessible • Perceived uneven surgeon quality • Decentralized decision making • No in-house space	• Single surgeon • Controversy surrounds surgery • Quality is questioned by some • Good mortality statistics • Relationships with referring physicians in question • Sense of continuous unrest
Anesthesia	• Cardiac trained • Nonrotating • System viewpoint	• Cardiac trained • Many rotate through service • Decentralized direction	• Cardiac trained • Many rotate through service • Decentralized direction
Support specialists	• High quality • Pulmonologist available	• High quality • No respiratory care department	• Well-regarded group • Stable
Nursing	• Physician directed • Specialty trained • Coordinated with team	• High-quality care • Strong on control • Obvious departmental barriers	• Lacks physician direction • Professional behavior is inconsistent • Quality is uneven • Lacks consistent motivation and training
Ancillary departments	• Coordinated • Patient driven • Efficient • Consultative	• Good • Team oriented • Consultative	• Adequate
Administration	• Program orientation • Involved • Facilitating and communicative • Risk active • Not control driven	• Well-intentioned • Lacks demonstrated commitment to program • Risk averse • Communicate inconsistently • Tend to polarize • Poor relations with nursing	• Well-intentioned strategically • Brilliant strategists • Weak on implementation • Control oriented

model program works diplomatically to preserve integrity among individual stakeholders. This is achieved in an environment in which it is understood that decisions are for the best interests of the *program*, not an individual or group.

Primary Care Physicians

The relationship with primary care physicians and medical groups has top priority in marketing efforts. Program planners recognize that, next to the patient, the primary care physician is the principal customer. An extensive network of primary care physicians is painstakingly maintained, and their loyalty is cultivated and nurtured.

Identity

Vigorous efforts are made to give the cardiovascular services product line the *identity* of an integrated program, even if the physical facilities do not lend themselves to such an identity. That is, the "program" may be spread over several facilities or medical groups, but the program identity rests with the physicians and the hospital that make up the program. Regular efforts are made to "spotlight" individuals within the various medical groups, thereby giving them a personal stake in the program and providing a resource to the community at large. Furthermore, a collaborative approach allows all participants to experience a sense of program ownership.

Decision Making

Many programs operate under a "benevolent dictator," a leader who, through force of personality and convention, can provide the program integration necessary for the consistent decision making that directs a program. In the absence of such an individual, a social process will be created that allows for consensus decision making, where a consensus becomes a *solution* with which no one disagrees, as opposed to a *compromise* in which everyone gives up something. The decision-making model implies that participants can generate a widespread program orientation that surpasses the self-centered decision making that routinely exists among related services.

Quality and Competence

The model cardiovascular program is built around highly competent physicians. However, what constitutes "highly competent" is vague and evolutionary in nature, with the market being the ultimate judge. Competent physicians, like leaders, demonstrate a variety of skills. Identifying a physician to lead the program is no easier than hiring clinical staff, drafting professional athletes, or selecting winning stocks.

This issue of competence affects the entire program and all participants. There is a focus on actively managing quality as a measure of competence in a collegial environment, where each person shares in ensuring high-quality care; that is not the conventional peer review environment. Quality management is seen by physicians as an asset, a way to improve not only the position of the cardiovascular program in the market, but also their individual and group positions within the program. (See chapter 5 for a more detailed discussion on the subject of quality management.)

Managed Care

In the model cardiovascular program, managed care is seen as an opportunity, not a threat, and managed care contracts are vigorously pursued with the posture of managing the environment rather than fighting or simply responding to it. In addition, a prevailing attitude among program staff is that the program and its management should be "on top of" everything, including local and regional developments in managed care. Every effort is made to be the market leader and to be innovative in response to developments in managed care and health service delivery systems.

Cost Orientation/Management

Historically, quality and cost in health care have been perceived as directly related. In the not-too-distant past, low cost seemed to imply low quality, and high cost seemed to promise high-quality care. However, in today's environment the model cardiovascular program is the low-cost leader because it provides high-quality, cost-effective care.

Certain markets not affected heavily by managed care may not realize as much benefit from low-cost leadership as those in a mature managed care market, but the pressure to deliver services profitably *and* competitively appears imminent for all programs. This is due to the growth of managed care and the continued focus of the federal Health Care Financing Administration (HCFA), which is contracting for "package-price" cardiovascular surgical services through their Demonstration Project in Cardiovascular Surgery.[3]

In the model program, the medical staff takes specific steps to manage case costs because doing so can increase the volume of business whereas failing to do so can lead to a decline. Rather than complaining of "cookbook medicine," program physicians insist on codifying their most efficient methods for patient care, and competition emerges among physicians in their efforts to lead the way in developing less costly patient care alternatives. These cost-effective patient care practices become the norm, with variations in the codified standard of practice identified and managed appropriately.

Growth

The staff is attentive to opportunities for growth along several spectrums — volume, technology, quality, market size, service capabilities, and so on. Opportunities may grow out of a program's competencies or be the impetus for a program to acquire additional resources and competencies.

Technology

Without being totally driven by technology, the model cardiovascular program seeks to maintain its position as a state-of-the-art program. Given the tremendous impact of technology on cardiovascular services in the recent past, managing technology will be critical to the development and restructuring of cardiovascular programs in the future.

The physicians in the model cardiovascular program indicate the need for new technology, recognize the resource limitations for acquiring certain technology (including staff and costs), and are judicious in the addition of technology. There is appreciation that technology not only is about equipment but about how one works; consequently, there is a focus on softer technologies as well as high-tech equipment.

Marketing

Marketing and promotion clearly play a role in the model program, but only as appropriate to the circumstance and the unique local market. They should not be overly relied on. Program participants recognize that the marketing of professional services is principally a matter of managing relationships with referring physicians and patients. Therefore, the marketing focus is on maintaining and developing the primary care network and is principally directed at physicians.

This is not to imply that other important target markets are ignored, particularly patients and payers, but acknowledgment that the physician market is the first line of support for a successful program. Promotion is carried out as a secondary marketing strategy to reinforce the management of relationships with referring physicians and the community. (Chapter 8 represents a full discussion of marketing plan development.)

Organization

Although a variety of support services can assist the model cardiovascular program, it is recognized within the hospital and by individual physicians as a separate contributing organization, "hospital within a hospital." Each physician, practice, staff member, and department treats the program as an entity and coordinates all of their efforts to benefit the program. The staff positions and their assigned activities constitute the key organizational elements of the program and support its day-to-day functions. Activities that are at odds with the program are quickly eliminated by program participants. If not managed appropriately, such independent programs can cause problems (for example, unproductive rivalries among services, departments, or programs). Managed appropriately, they can become powerful forces within the organization. Key organizational elements of a model program are discussed in detail in the next sections. Further information on organizing a cardiovascular program is provided in chapter 5.

The model organizational elements that follow elaborate on the matrix in figure 4-7. They reflect the seven most prominent departments or services comprising the full-service CV program. The model described is based on a community hospital-based, moderate-size program that performs 200–500 cardiovascular surgeries, 800–2,000 cardiac catheterizations, and 200–400 interventional procedures per year.

Again, the model is intended as an example only. Model program components must be accepted by participants as part of the planning process.

Cardiology

Cardiology in the model program typically is represented by a variety of groups and solo practitioners but is distinguished by one dominant group. Despite challenge from one or more competing groups over time, it is clear that this dominant group provides the principal direction for cardiology. The cardiology group performs no general internal medicine and is based on the hospital's campus. Depending on local conditions and the existence of strong competing groups with significant market share, cardiology may have special relationships in the emergency room and the noninvasive laboratory (although typically not exclusive of other primary cardiology players). A medical director oversees cardiology and related activities.

Cardiovascular Surgery

Generally, the model program is served by a single group of cardiovascular surgeons who have strong relationships within their group and are management oriented. The group is very aggressive in the managed care arena, and individuals within the group recognize that case cost management is a key factor in the competitive environment. Cardiovascular surgeons take active interest in case costs and regularly address the issue of standard treatment protocols (STPs), actively involving cardiologists who refer cases to them.

Cardiovascular surgeons are accessible to cardiologists for collaborative decision making and make a concerted effort to see that all patients return to the primary care physician who referred the case. They also maintain regular contact with the physician during the course of care.

Cardiac Anesthesia

Cardiac anesthesia is provided by experienced anesthesiologists with specialized training who are dedicated to cardiac surgery to the extent that economics allow it. They are involved closely in the care of postoperative patients to ensure continuity of care.

Support Specialists

Strong consulting support is available from the pulmonary medicine, infectious disease, neurology, nephrology, pathology, and radiology staffs. These consultants have some specialized knowledge of CV surgery as it relates to their areas of interest.

Nursing

A strong relationship exists between the nursing units and the operating room staff. Nurses in the cardiac surgery intensive care unit care exclusively for cardiac patients and have specialized training. The nursing staff is patient oriented and physician oriented and provides an important link among the various physicians involved in patient care. Cardiac nurses have participated actively in the development of STPs and manage their nursing care on these consensus-based standards.

Ancillary Departments

Ancillary departments — respiratory care, physical therapy, dietary, and so on — are familiar with the unique needs of cardiovascular patients and are patient oriented. The hospital-based physicians associated with ancillary departments cooperate with the CV program and are readily available for consultation.

Administration

The hospital administrative and management staff is program oriented, regardless of the organizational structure. They see the program as an essential hospital service and work consistently to further its purposes. They promote communication and are not control oriented so that the program can move aggressively, internally and externally.

Elements of a Successful Cardiovascular Program Strategy

As stated early in this chapter, strategy must be simple without being simplistic. In large organizations, elaborate strategies usually are not adopted easily because, among other things, they cannot be communicated effectively to the number of individuals needed to ensure their success. Generally, successful program development strategies will be built around these elements: medical staff, mission, market, and management. The vision will take into account all of these strategic themes.

Medical Staff

In professional sports, the franchise must be built around the players; all of an owner's elaborate efforts cannot produce a successful team without quality players. So it is in hospital management. Disconcerting as it may be to administrators and managers, the truth is that what the hospital controls *least* matters the *most*. That is, *successful programs are built around successful physicians*. Recognizing this is the most important lesson in formulating successful strategy. The next most important lesson is that what is deemed successful today may not hold for tomorrow; thus success is dynamic and requires constant effort. As the cardiovascular services market becomes increasingly crowded and competitive, these lessons will hold true even more.

Mission Statement

Mission, interpreted as vision, will differentiate successful programs from struggling programs. As physicians and managers collaborate to articulate their vision for the program, it will gain in strength to face future challenges. Furthermore, this collaboration will lead to integration of physician and program goals, resulting in closer partnerships. This goal alignment will be the product of identifying external threats from a changing environment and realizing opportunities for physician and program managers. The threats will be mitigated more successfully and the opportunities realized more routinely as a result of this integration.

Market Changes

Successful program management will respond and adapt to the changing marketplace. For example, the creative planning team that seeks opportunities with managed care groups and physician partnerships rather than deal with them purely as competitors for patients is adapting, not reacting, to change. As seen in chapter 3, change will be evident in demographics, the regulatory environment, the managed care industry, demand for various procedures, and the influence of accelerated competition.

Management

Although the medical staff is central to program development, inspired management leadership will be crucial in the future competitive arena. This leadership must be physician centered to provide the proper environment in which to develop physician direction, remove obstacles from physicians' paths, and create the proper forum for program development. For example, although managers control technology, marketing, facilities, staffing, and so forth, they do not usurp cardiovascular physicians' principal relationship with referring physicians and patients.

Summary

Strategy is a structure for thinking about the future of a program and the external variables that will affect it and the internal variables that will be key to its survival and success. This framework of ideas leads to the development of a programmatic vision that guides the formation of a value system, which in turn leads to the convictions and objectives necessary to make congruent decisions.

Strategy involves the process of organizing actions in order to accomplish agreed-upon group outcomes. Strategy is built in part around the comparison of where the program would like to be (the model program) and where it presently is. Bridging these gaps and exploiting gaps identified in the competition is the principal method for formulating strategy. Because visions and strategies must ultimately be simple enough to be communicated without being simplistic, a concerted effort must be made to translate the strategy into as few statements and concepts as possible. Identifying the barriers and gateways to success and limiting them to no more than a dozen issues and actions will accomplish this objective. Successful strategy will be tied to successfully integrating the medical staff, management, mission, and the market.

☐ *References*

1. Bennis, W., and Nauus, B. *Leaders: The Strategies for Taking Charge.* New York City: Harper and Row Publishers, 1985.

2. Steiner, G. *Strategic Planning: What Every Manager Must Know.* New York City: The Free Press, 1979.

3. Tokarski, C. Bypass surgery targeted for pricing test. *Modern Healthcare* 21(5):3, Feb. 4, 1991.

Chapter 5

Program Management

Management is a process of moving a group toward the accomplishment of a common objective. Human groups have developed generally along the lines of a hierarchy that provides for the performance of management functions by a subset of the larger group. This chapter outlines the five broad areas of the management process as they relate to cardiovascular services:

1. Principles of organization
2. Functions of management (planning and setting goals, making decisions, directing, exerting control, organizing)
3. Management approaches (product line management, cardiovascular product line inventory, medical direction, linking programs, joint ventures and other expansion strategies)
4. Cardiovascular services management and staffing
5. Managing cardiovascular information and quality

Much of the discussion refers to generic organizations, which allows easier application of the concepts to the various organizations involved in the delivery of cardiovascular services (including the cardiovascular program itself, individual departments within the program, the entire hospital, physician groups, and so on).

Principles of Organization

A cardiovascular program is a social organization in which successful management involves application of a variety of fundamental organizational concepts. Sociology and psychology play a role in these concepts. The following discussion outlines some basic principles of organizations.

Every group has a purpose, an objective it seeks to accomplish. This objective is understood to differing degrees by members of the group, and differences often exist in their interpretation of the group's purpose. Organizations can be unstructured and informal, such as a group of medical colleagues, or they can be structured and formal, such as a hospital. However, every group or organization has *boundaries* that define who is in the group or organization.

Organizations take on a life of their own; that is, they are made up of people, not buildings or equipment. Consequently, the organization changes slowly over time through the addition and subtraction of people. For instance, the resignation of one part-time nurse in a cardiac catheterization unit changes the organization. This recognition of the human factor is a principle critical to successful management; to speak of "the organization" is to refer to *a certain group of people who come together for the purpose of accomplishing an agreed-on set of tasks.* Knowing this principle, then, is the first step toward moving an organization forward.

As the organization matures, it begins to establish *values* and *norms* for members' behavior. It then defines *roles* for all of its members. Most organizations are modeled on a hierarchy that establishes *authority* within the organization.

Organizational behavior can become complex, especially if it is understood that every organization exists as a *system* or a subset of a larger system and that every system generally "houses" smaller systems. For example, the surgery and cardiology departments are organizations embedded in (are subsets in) the larger hospital organization. The hospital is a subset of a larger system, perhaps a multihospital system, the community, the state, and the health care industry. Conversely, the surgery and cardiology departments house smaller systems such as the cardiovascular surgery team, cardiac catheterization staff, transcription staff, and so forth. Organizational flowcharts help identify areas and functions and describe how authority flows and decisions are made.

Hospitals are made more complex because of the presence of the medical staff, whose legal obligations, independent mode of operation, and relationship to the hospital create many of the challenges faced by hospital management. As a rule, physicians are independent contractors and therefore seek benefits for themselves as smaller organizations. At the same time, many physicians are affiliated with hospitals whose objectives are so similar to their own—although never precisely the same—that the physicians function more like hospital employees than members of the medical staff. In short, the medical staff is not easily categorized and dealt with as a group. Rather, the membership role of each physician or each medical group within the hospital organization must be determined individually.

A cardiovascular program is even more complex because typically it involves not only a different set of boundaries but boundaries that often do not conform to the formal parameters created by the hospital or the medical staff. Successful cardiovascular programs have resolved the issues of program boundaries, either directly or indirectly, by these specific accomplishments:

- They created a legitimate method for determining which physicians are included within the boundaries.
- They developed effective modifications to the hospital's formal structure to accommodate the program's need for specific management.
- They defined unique norms and values for the program through the involvement of strong physicians. This results in medical direction that allows for clear objective setting, efficiency, and effectiveness in the use of resources and decision making that properly positions a clinical program in a competitive market.

Planning and Setting Goals

Although organizational behavior is goal directed, goals sometimes become vague and lose their force, thereby creating confusion within a program. Despite feeling the effects of this confusion, organization members cannot see uncertainty of purpose as the cause. Largely this is because individuals are more interested in achieving their personal goals. Therefore, when organizational agendas become sidetracked members fill the void with their personal goals — even if those goals differ from those of others in the organization. For example, whereas many cardiovascular programs state increased market share or enhanced customer satisfaction as their goals, individual stakeholders might have different goals (an employee might want more compensation, an invasive cardiologist might want to perform more catheterizations, or a cardiovascular surgeon might want more time off). Sometimes the goals are altruistic (a teaching physician wishing to expand a university hospital's cardiovascular research capacities or a staff member wishing to include inner-city areas on a mobile cardiac laboratory route).

Although these goals are not necessarily mutually exclusive of organizational goals, they are different; and this "goal incongruity" produces individual actions that can defeat the purposes of the organization as well as the purposes of other members of the organization. To the extent that an organization can clarify its mission, it can bring about *goal congruity* with its members. *Finding the mechanisms to reconcile differences among goals is a key function of the management team.* Goal congruity among key constituencies allows a cardiovascular program to become more effective in attaining its stated goals.

On an operational or departmental level, managers generally develop broad and attainable *goals* and specific *objectives* that are attainable and time targeted. Each objective is accompanied by an action plan that specifies completion date and assigns responsibility for completion. These goals, objectives, and action plans should conform to the strategy identified for the cardiovascular program. (As discussed in chapter 4, planning and strategy formulation determine what ends the organization is seeking. Strategy development for cardiovascular programs includes formulating policy, crafting strategy, and determining tactics.)

In many cases, goals and objectives will be completed in conjunction with a hospitalwide objective-setting process. As part of the planning process the hospital will determine both the format for presentation of objectives and the schedule for their implementation. (*Strategic Thinking: New Frontier for Hospital Management,* by James B. Webber and Joseph P. Peters, is an excellent guide to the planning process.[1])

Making Decisions

Goals and objectives are the raw material of decision making, the most important function of management and the function that separates managers from the rest of the organization. After alternatives are identified and evaluated, management makes a decision based on the likelihood that the alternative chosen will achieve the desired result.

Decision making is so much a part of the management process that it easily is taken for granted. Generally decisions are divided into two types: routine and nonroutine.

Routine decisions are made in the general conduct and transaction of regular business. Examples include arranging the staffing schedule and re-ordering supplies at specified times and in predetermined quantities. Systems should be established to delegate these routine decisions as far down the organization as possible. Not only does this enhance the quality of the decision, it enhances the self-esteem and organizational involvement of the decision maker.

Policies and procedures are routine decisions written for the hospital and for individual departments. Policies are *guides to thinking,* whereas procedures are *guides to action.* Hospitalwide manuals usually address policies, whereas departmental manuals focus more on procedures that guide the activities of departmental personnel. For example, a hospitalwide policy might dictate that every employee is entitled to a specified amount of paid time off, thereby guiding institutional thinking on the subject of paid time off. The hospitalwide procedure, on the other hand, will outline exactly how paid time off is calculated and recorded, which is action oriented. Similarly, departmental policy will direct that paid time off can be taken only at the discretion and convenience of the department, and departmental procedure specifies how and when requests for time off must be made.

Nonroutine decisions occur less frequently and are more difficult to pre-program. For example, selection of major catheterization equipment or implementation of a new surgery scheduling system cannot be decided at lower levels of the organization; nor can the criteria for making such decisions be predetermined. Although nonroutine decisions also should be delegated to the extent possible, generally they require higher-level involvement because they have to do with making policy. Some nonroutine decisions, such as selection of major equipment, will require an application of creativity or knowledge not required in lower levels of the organization. Other nonroutine decisions (for example, modification of the surgery scheduling system) are political in nature and require extra communication and negotiation to "sell" the decision. Understanding that different conditions demand different treatment is helpful in planning organizational activities and improving the quality of decisions.

All decisions are evaluated along two dimensions: *quality* and *acceptance*. The type of decision (command, consensus, consultative, or convenience) will dictate which decision-making process is used. For example, a *command decision* emphasizes the quality of the decision; a *consensus decision* emphasizes acceptance. In some cases, quality and acceptance are equally important, resulting in a *consultative decision,* whereas a decision for which neither is important is a *convenience decision.*

Setting objectives and making decisions can be more difficult in health care organizations compared with non–health care organizations – especially for cardiovascular services. As discussed earlier in this chapter, organizations have permeable boundaries. Many cardiovascular programs have poorly defined boundaries, particularly with respect to physician participants. Cardiologists affiliated at more than one hospital must be considered a legitimate part of the organization; yet, unlike cardiologists affiliated exclusively with the hospital or the cardiovascular surgery team contracted exclusively with the hospital, they often are not treated as full members. Clearly, the goals of the "exclusives" more closely parallel those of the hospital and the cardiovascular program. Politics, then, can be a barrier to setting goals and making decisions in a cardiovascular program.

Program management (which includes physicians) decisions are enhanced if it is clear who can participate in the objective-setting process and who has specialized knowledge to help assess the environment. Frequently, the authority structure accountable for decision making is also poorly defined. This creates an environment in which decision makers are reluctant to accept the risk for what could be good decisions. For example, package pricing for cardiovascular services involves combining the hospital's charges with the physician's fees. Because of the number of participants – cardiologists, cardiovascular surgeons, cardiac anesthesiologists, and hospital-based physicians – arriving at the final price is a complex process. Each participant must accept some risk for the consequences of the pricing decision. Determining who will be included in the package is, therefore, a difficult task.

Objectives of program managers can conflict with those of the hospital, just as objectives of program participants (physicians and staff) can be incongruent with those of program managers. Although no one entity is always "correct," the organization must build measures into its structure to avoid or resolve conflict.

Directing

Directing, which involves guiding or steering the organization and its staff, is a function of leadership. There are different styles of directing: dictatorial, autocratic, modified democratic, or laissez faire. Each style is effective in particular situations and at specific times. Directing also involves taking action, supervising and prioritizing others' activities while at the same time moving the organization toward its goals.

Unfortunately, many health care organizations suffer poor leadership, particularly by physicians. John Gardner, former secretary of the (then) Department of Health, Education and Welfare and author of many insightful books on leadership, has identified 10 tasks of leadership:[2]

1. Envisioning goals
2. Affirming values
3. Regenerating values
4. Motivating
5. Managing
6. Achieving unity
7. Explaining
8. Serving as symbol
9. Representing
10. Renewing

Fostering physician leadership means more than occasionally soliciting physicians' opinions. Leadership involves the whole person, including vision, values, integrity, and charisma. Furthermore, it assumes a consistent role within the organization that allows the expression of power, influence, and authority. Leadership is also a behavior pattern that stems from convictions, loyalty, and an emphasis on goals, on the program, and on the inherent importance of successfully managing relationships with a variety of publics.

Resolving conflict is an essential management skill. Conflicts emerge from a variety of sources and, according to Alan C. Filley,[3] involve either competitive conflict in which the parties strive to win or disruptive conflict in which the parties strive to defeat one another.

Consensus-building and problem-solving behavior are strategies used to avoid or resolve conflict. Consensus building results in a resolution to which no one objects. This differs from a compromise, where everyone gives up something. Problem-solving behavior focuses on defeating the *problem* rather than another party; it avoids voting, seeks facts, accepts conflict philosophically, and avoids personality clashes.

Exerting Control

Despite its negative connotation, control is a management style used by many people. Control does not imply regulating behavior per se but accomplishing objectives. Exerting control relies on monitoring progress being made toward goal fulfillment. Progress is measured using four parameters:

1. A standard or output goal
2. A mechanism for measuring current activity
3. A methodology for comparing current activity with the standard or goal
4. A means for communicating and correcting shortcomings[4]

Specific behaviors are problems *only* to the extent that they prevent objectives from being achieved. "End orientation," as opposed to "means orientation," which is more restrictive, is essential to building a vital organization. Control, then, measures current activities against predetermined goals, compares the results, and initiates appropriate remedies.

Several common control mechanisms, in place at most hospitals, will affect a cardiovascular program. These systems include budgeting, budget variance reporting, service unit forecasting, and employee evaluations. More and more the control function focuses not on inputs to the system (budgets) but on outputs; hence, the emphasis on quality and quality management systems.

Organizing

Organizing involves structuring the components, relationships, or tasks so that efficient relationships are established to process the work necessary to conduct business.

In the past few years, cardiovascular services have been developed and organized with cardiac surgery as the centerpiece. Surgical orientation was appropriate, given the focus of resources and the dominance of surgical approaches in the treatment of cardiovascular disease.

Clearly this focus has moved into the catheterization laboratory and, therefore, into the realm of cardiologists. This change in focus is mainly due to technological advances and the growing influence of primary care in delivery systems. Because cardiologists are closer to the primary care (that is, primary physician) level and have a longer relationship with cardiac patients than do cardiovascular surgeons (whose involvement is episodic), cardiologists have become more influential in patient care and in managing relationships with primary care physicians, medical groups, and payers.

Organizing and ensuring the success of a cardiovascular program is made easier with strong medical direction. In the typical hospital organization, the cardiology department reports to the vice-president of clinical/professional services, and cardiovascular surgery reports to the vice-president for patient/ nursing services. In some organizations, both groups report to the same individual, which improves program integration but may result in conflicts between the operating room and the nursing units. Regardless of reporting relationships, cooperation and coordination between the two departments can be strained.

Heightened status of the cardiologist in the delivery system affects a number of organizations and organizational structures. Whereas the cardiac surgeon — and therefore the operating room — heretofore has dominated the administrative structure, the cardiology department is emerging as the primary entity. This change is occurring in part because the cardiology manager is devoted to the cardiology product line while the operating room manager responds to multiple product lines. Although in many operating rooms one supervisor may focus on CV surgery, there generally is an additional level of organization between that supervisor and top-level administration. Certainly operating room personnel could manage the service, but their multiple loyalties affect their ability to fill the role effectively.

As cardiology managers (who are typically cardiovascular technicians or cardiac catheterization nurses with advanced management training) continue to influence the organization, their professional affiliations (the American College of Cardiovascular Administrators, or ACCA) gain in importance. Currently no formal credentialing or training program exists for these managers; but with the growing demand for their expertise, organizations such as the ACCA provide education, networking opportunities, and program standardization.

Although one management structure will predominate, this will not eliminate the potential for fragmentation of principal services. Therefore, product or service line management is an alternative structure in many organizations.

Product Line Management

For CV services a product line management (PLM) approach, as defined in chapter 1, will not improve on incompetent management, nor will it overcome strong divisional rivalries within the organization. The difference in results is not due to the method of implementation or the system used, but rather the individuals involved, especially the physicians.

Organizations of the medical staff involved in the product line must be structured so that PLM is responsive to their practice patterns and unique personalities. Further, PLM is not an "easy answer" to difficult organizational or market-based problems.

No single organizational structure fits every situation. As always, success will be the result of strong leadership, hard work, and timely decision making.

To provide the necessary focus for the cardiovascular services program, many organizations institute a hybrid of product line management and traditional departmental structure. In well-managed organizations, a responsibility allocation system will evolve, in which key administrative personnel assume principal authority and responsibility for cardiovascular services. The result is a *matrix* organization, in which the functional responsibility for individual departments remains intact, but the programmatic responsibility falls to different members of the administrative staff.

A matrix organization is simple to implement and effective in that it requires the support of the highest levels in the organization, who guarantee participation by their respective departments. This structure eliminates many of the authority issues that follow direct development of PLM. Further, it allows physicians to address their programmatic concerns with top-level administrators and to identify opportunities cooperatively. Over time, a matrix organization can evolve into a workable service line program. Ultimately, each program will evolve its own organizational structure in response to the size of the hospital, the size of the program, the demands of the environment, and the capabilities of the individuals involved.

Cardiovascular Product Line Inventory

A cardiovascular product line inventory (see sample in table 5-1) is valuable in assessing services currently available within a cardiovascular program and can be used as a planning document to identify missing programs or services. (A similar document can be used in the competitor assessment process, discussed in chapter 3, to document services available in the community and to identify market niches.)

The cardiovascular product line inventory is arrayed around seven categories: management, intake, evaluation, therapy, care, rehabilitation/ follow-up, and education. Each category is then divided into general services and product line services. By distinguishing between services currently available and those planned, the product line inventory becomes a helpful planning tool for cardiovascular product line development.

Table 5-1. Cardiovascular Product Line Inventory

Management	Intake	Evaluation	Therapy	Care	Rehabilitation/Follow-up	Education
• CEO	• Medical staff	• Laboratory	• Medications/pharmokinetics	• Nursing services	• Home health	• Wellness
• Senior vice-president and COO	• Emergency department	• Radiology	• Surgery	• M/S beds	• Social services	• Community education
• VP—professional services	• Transfers from other hospitals	• Nuclear medicine	• Pulmonary	• Intensive care:	• Cardiopulmonary rehabilitation	• In-service education
• VP—nursing services	• Physician referral service	• Neurophysiology (NCV/EEG/EMG)	• PT/OT	ICU	• Patient representative	• Continuing medical education
• Critical care supervisor	• Ambulatory care center	• Respiratory care	• Blood bank	CCU	• Vascular rehabilitation	• Enhanced physical training
• Administrative director/operations	• HMO contracts	• MRI	• IV therapy	• SNF facility	• Lipid clinic	• Staff training for outlying hospital staffs and physicians' office staffs
• VP—marketing	• Urgent care center	• CT	• Physical therapy/rehabilitation	• CCU		• Increased community CV education
• Marketing coordinator	• Cardiology department	• EKG	• Thrombolytic therapy	• Radio-monitored telemetry beds		• Enhanced and comprehensive CV education for technical and clinical staff
• Manager—diagnostic imaging (cardiac catheterization)	• Catheterization laboratory	• Stress testing	• Pacemakers	• Cardiovascular patient unit		
• Chairperson—department of internal medicine	• Internists	• Cardiac ultrasound	• PTCA (angioplasty)	• Intermediate acuity nursing unit (step-down)		
• CV services director	• GP/FPs	• Holter monitoring	• CV surgery	• CSICU		
• Manager—cardiology laboratory	• Cardiologist	• Catheterization				
• Supervisor—CCU, CV surgery	• CV surgeon	• Nuclear cardiology				
• Medical directors	• Cardiac anesthesiologists	• Cardiac ultrasound (echocardiography)				
—Cardiologist	• Primary care network	• Joint-ventured noninvasive laboratory				
—Cath lab	• Mobile screening					
—Cardiac rehab						
—CV surgery						
• Cardiac coordinators						

When appropriate, each entry in the product line inventory can be expanded into a schedule of program development so as to prioritize opportunities based on variables such as program components, market served, facilities required, and staffing issues.

Medical Direction

Although strong physician leadership cannot be manufactured, it is essential that the issue of medical direction be assessed properly before making any decisions about how to organize the cardiovascular program. Hospitals tend to use administrative management to compensate for lack of physician leadership. Although this may be a reasonable intention, it will work only where there is little or no competition or where physicians are willing to be led *as a group* by management and to agree generally on issues presented to them. In both situations, strong and visionary management will be required for this strategy to be successful.

Absent proper medical direction, confusion and disagreement over program goals lead to poorly defined program direction, which in turn breeds discontent and disillusionment. This is particularly the case where there is competition for cardiovascular patients and where the competition demonstrates strong medical direction. Without proper medical direction, all attempts to bring about meaningful change or to improve market position will meet with limited success at best.

Another way to achieve proper medical direction is to reorganize the medical community (for example, forming a cardiology group where previously there were solo practitioners or small groups). Where possible, solutions must build on the existing medical community or at least grow out of a consensus within the medical community.

Linking Programs

Several cardiovascular programs have been strategically linked with other clinical programs including vascular services, pulmonary medicine, circulatory services, or other hospitals. Such linkages offer definite benefits from the standpoint of resource allocation and may represent promotional and marketing opportunities as well.

Service linkage sounds appealing, especially when developing a "circulatory institute," which appears more inclusive, compared to forming a cardiovascular program. However, considered from the standpoint of the marketplace, a circulatory institute may be impractical, even disadvantageous. A circulatory institute, while more comprehensive than a cardiovascular program, may not attract cardiac patients. Potential patients view their problem as a heart problem, not a circulation problem.

Market research can determine whether there is value to be gained from such packaging from the standpoint of the consumer or payer communities. The medical staff will generally be reluctant to bring these specialties together. Absent any obvious benefits or opportunities, such combinations should be avoided; advantages to the program must flow from value to the participating clinicians. The collaboration of cardiovascular services with vascular or pulmonary medicine may result in the perception on the part of physicians that there is a lack of focus or some confusion in the political dynamics that have manifested themselves historically in these areas.

Joint Ventures and Other Opportunities for Expansion

Joint ventures should not be overlooked in considering ways to develop a cardiovascular program. Joint ventures can involve other hospitals as well as physicians. Much has been written about joint venturing, and because the legal environment for joint ventures is changing rapidly, the comments here include a range of possibilities. (Note: The joint venture opportunities here are for illustrative purposes only and under no circumstances should be substituted for competent legal advice.)

Because noninvasive services routinely are available in cardiologists' offices, joint venture opportunities are limited among cardiologists. Hospitals in medical communities that have not added these services should test the feasibility of such joint ventures with cardiologists. In addition to a simple echocardiography equipment venture, consideration should be given to developing a more extensive cardiac diagnostic center and, in certain settings, to forming a mobile noninvasive cardiology service. Noninvasive vascular laboratories should also be investigated.

The number of invasive cardiology procedures recently has been on the rise. This is due to two factors: Medicare's decision to reimburse facility fees for non–hospital-based catheterization laboratories and increased safety of catheterization. Assessment of freestanding and mobile catheterization laboratory development is appropriate for joint venturers such as development/ service companies and larger hospitals.

Two other joint venture possibilities are cardiac rehabilitation, which requires at least one committed cardiologist to oversee program development, and cardiac screening programs.

Managing

Management will need to be evaluated in terms of capability and availability. Adding a dedicated catheterization laboratory will mean the addition of a manager, whereas managing a joint-use room falls directly to the radiology manager. The addition of cardiovascular surgery will increase the volume of activity in the catheterization laboratory to a level where a manager will be required, and an operating room staff member will be elevated to the position of cardiovascular surgery supervisor. Only large programs have dedicated cardiac surgery managers. In general, the cardiac surgery intensive care unit functions best as a separate unit under the direct supervision of a CSICU manager, who typically has two to four years of training and experience in CSICU nursing.

Management, like other disciplines, has built up a system of principles that guide management behavior. Ten of these principles are outlined below:

1. An individual's responsibility cannot be delegated to someone else.
2. Authority should be delegated as far into the organization as possible.
3. Authority must be sufficient to allow fulfillment of the responsibility.
4. Levels of authority should be limited.
5. Clear lines of authority should be established.
6. No one should report to more than one authority and all staff must know to whom they report.
7. Expectations of each individual should be defined.
8. The number of positions reporting to a single individual should be limited.
9. The organization should be kept simple.
10. The organization should be kept flexible.

These principles apply to every organization and can be used by the cardiovascular administrator or manager to enhance the effectiveness of the program.

Staffing

Whereas organizing involves the structuring of functions, staffing involves selecting and organizing people to perform job functions. The staffing plan developed for cardiovascular services depends partly on local practices and preferences as well as on assumptions about volume, both initially and over the first several months of the program.

The basic staff required for a diagnostic cardiac catheterization laboratory consists of one registered nurse, one certified radiologic technologist, and one cardiovascular technologist. Cardiac catheterization laboratories can be developed in connection with an existing or newly added general angiographic suite (for circulatory or cardiac X ray) within the radiology department. Staffing for such a joint-use room can include existing personnel. For example, the registered nurse and the cardiovascular technologist may be trained from current hospital personnel. The certified radiologic technologist would probably come from the existing radiology staff.

A cardiac catheterization laboratory registered nurse must be licensed as a registered nurse and have basic cardiac life support (BCLS) certification and certification in countershock (use of defibrillation equipment). The certifications are required by the Joint Commission on Accreditation of Healthcare Organizations (JCAHO). It is recommended that critical care registered nurse (CCRN) certification, advanced cardiac life support (ACLS) certification, and comprehensive experience in a cardiac catheterization laboratory be considered as optimal qualifications for this position.

The certified radiologic technologist should have a valid state CRT certificate, and the JCAHO requires BCLS certification. Here again, it is advisable that the technologist have experience in angiographic procedures, specifically cardiac catheterization, and have a knowledge of cinemographic equipment, development of cine film, and quality standards as they relate to cardiac catheterization laboratory functioning.

Generally, the cardiovascular technologist is not required to have state certification, but professional society registry or eligibility for registry examinations can be an evaluation criterion. In addition to the BCLS certification required by the JCAHO, it is advisable that this individual have extensive experience in the cardiac catheterization laboratory, particularly physiologic monitoring and recording procedures and certification in countershock.

Obviously, the addition of cardiovascular surgery is much more complex and from a staffing perspective will have ramifications throughout the institution. In addition to having direct impacts on the operating room and the CSICU, it will affect several clinical departments: pharmacy, respiratory therapy, physical therapy, noninvasive cardiology, and nuclear medicine, for example.

Within the operating room, the basic team required to staff cardiovascular surgery and to support the operating team includes the following:

- One extracorporeal perfusion specialist (perfusionist). Perfusionists may be hired by the hospital, employed by the surgeon, or brought to the hospital under contract with a perfusion company. In any case, the perfusionist should be board certified as a clinical perfusionist by a recognized certification agency.
- Two cardiovascular ICU registered nurses. Cardiovascular surgical nurses are required to have a valid state license as well as BCLS certification. It is strongly recommended that ACLS certification and comprehensive training and experience in cardiovascular surgery nursing be considered essential for these positions. Where available, nurses with CCRN certification and ACLS certification as well as comprehensive training and postoperative cardiovascular surgical nursing are recommended. Given the acuity level of postoperative patients, a one-

to-one nurse–patient ratio is required. When starting a new program, strong surgical nurses can be sent to training programs under the direction of the surgeon.

- One perfusion assistant.
- One surgical technician.

Access to cardiac rehabilitation must be provided, either directly or by referral. Cardiac rehabilitation departments require a cardiac rehabilitation nurse specialist and physical therapists. Some programs include an exercise physiologist in the staff mix to supervise patient exercise activities. It is also recommended that a consulting dietitian, a patient education registered nurse, and a social worker be considered part of the cardiac rehabilitation team, in order to reinforce necessary life-style changes among patients and to arrange for necessary community-based services.

Managing Information

Information plays an important role from the systems perspective that the purpose of organizations is to attain group goals and that the function of management is to direct the actions of the organization. Information is essentially the feedback an organization receives regarding its success in moving the organization toward its goals.

It is important to differentiate between *data* and *information,* particularly given the overabundance of "input" in our computerized world. Data are the raw material from which information is drawn. For information to be readily available, a *data system* must be in place. A data system will:

- Classify
- Collect
- Calculate
- Communicate
- Record
- Reproduce
- Retrieve
- Store
- Sort

A telephone book is a good example of a data system in that it allows the user to perform all of the above functions. A telephone book is not an *information system* because it deals only with data.

Information can be differentiated from data in that information is:

- Accurate
- Timely

- Relevant
- Concise
- Complete

In the context of the management function, data become information only after meeting the criteria listed above *and* after being used to make decisions.

Based on the preceding, a management information system is best understood as *a set of interrelated parts brought together for the purpose of extracting information from data for use in making decisions by management in their effort to move the organization toward the accomplishment of its objectives.*

Because information technology is changing so rapidly, it is important to focus on system attributes and outcome expectations rather than on system specifications. Program managers will continue to receive data from the financial system regarding their financial performance, budget variance reports, and a variety of statistical data. The marketing and planning functions will continue to assist in the provision of market share data, certain competitor data, and so forth. Many techniques will be used to survey the environment for such changes and the evolution of the regulatory system, changes in technology, modifications of the reimbursement mechanisms, and so on. Many of these data defy organization, but the interested manager will develop mechanisms to ensure that these sources are accessed regularly.

Systems can be devised to manage the program on a daily basis. The program's product will be refined and defined regularly, including descriptions of the DRGs involved, procedures performed, services provided, markets served, physicians involved, and so on. Other data sources will be developed and expanded over time.

The program should provide regular access to the following specific information:

- Patient information
  - Demographics
  - Account and record numbers
  - Admission and discharge data
- Clinical measures
  - Diagnoses
  - Procedures
  - Severity indicators and measures
  - Length of stay
  - Charge and resource consumption
- Payer data
- Billing data
- Physician roster
- Physician utilization results

- Staffing
- Managed care roster
- Quality indicators
- Physician referral sources
- Patient satisfaction
- Referring physician satisfaction

These data elements will be useful in management's efforts to enhance financial performance, improve productivity, reduce case costs, improve and maintain quality, enhance patient satisfaction, expand referring physician satisfaction, increase referral sources, and so on.

Managing Quality

As already noted, competition will focus increasingly on quality and cost, as is true in any mature market (see chapter 6 for a discussion on cost management). Therefore, in the future one of the most important aspects of management for cardiovascular programs will be quality management. In the 1980s, health care observers spoke somewhat passively of quality using terms such as *quality assurance,* but the language has become much stronger and more action oriented toward quality as a strategic imperative.

The high value placed on quality in health care is implicit in the Hippocratic oath and in the very notion of professionalism. Requiring as it does advanced training and skills, the term *professionalism* implies the attribute of quality. Each health care profession has evolved its own code of ethics that not only embody values in support of quality, but create a professional identity based on shared training and ability, which are used to comfort if not cure the sick. Application of special knowledge and skills to improve the lot of the client not only is the key to all professions but, arguably, is one definition of *quality.*

Until recently in the United States, organized efforts to ensure quality in health care were largely voluntary. The Flexner Report of 1910 brought to public notice the sorry state of medical education and, by extension, the quality of physicians.[5] The Joint Commission on Accreditation of Hospitals (now known as the Joint Commission on Accreditation of Healthcare Organizations) began providing voluntary accreditation to hospitals until the advent of Medicare, when reimbursement to hospitals was linked to accreditation status. As government funding of health care has grown, so have regulation, inspection, licensing, and consumer protection measures, all in support of quality in the provision of health care services by professionals and institutions.

The history of quality management in hospitals has been one of successive levels of requirements by regulatory agencies and an often confusing succession of terms for measuring and ensuring quality of care. What was once known as "quality assurance" gave way to "quality review," which brought with it an emphasis on monitoring and evaluation of clinical activities and an array of standards to be met. Sometimes providers were uncertain as to how specific standards were to be achieved. The current accepted terminology within health care organizations is *total quality management* and *continuous quality improvement,* implying ongoing application of quality standards, constant feedback, and continuous improvement of the product and work processes.

Accelerated competition in health care, not only among hospitals but also among hospitals and urgent care centers, freestanding diagnostic and treatment centers, and private physicians' offices, has forced hospital executives to look for new management models that will ensure survival of their institutions. Changes in government reimbursement and the growth of managed care as a model for much health care in the United States have only served to increase the challenge for hospitals to increase the quality of care and decrease the cost of care, or to cease operations.

In a field that only recently acknowledged its role as a service industry, the notion of competition for patients and good physicians not only has been unwelcome but distasteful to many executives, trustees, and medical staff members. Hospitals are complex, hierarchical organizations staffed by a highly structured matrix of professionals dominated by physicians who value their professional autonomy. Consequently, physicians, nurses, social workers, and other professionals have been socialized in the structured, status-conscious, and nonegalitarian world of hospitals.

Most hospitals resist seeing health care as a service industry much like hotels and airlines. For example, the concept of customer satisfaction, long a key indicator of corporate quality in the service industries and now a measure of hospital quality, is in direct conflict with traditional notions of medical specialization, professional dominance, and patient passivity. However, forward-looking hospital executives have begun to look to other industries for models of management and quality improvement that are adaptable to health care organizations.

Some of the most popular and effective industry models were initially successful in service industries and in manufacturing companies. Many of the most enduring have been learned from the Japanese manufacturing industries. Theorists such as W. Edwards Deming,[6] Joseph Juran,[7] and Philip Crosby[8] have advanced techniques of quality improvement that have contributed to progress in health care organizations. Even the JCAHO has synthesized and translated its theories for use in health care organizations.[9] An example is the JCAHO's recent emphasis on the process of quality management as opposed to the structural approach favored in the past.

The most significant theories include the importance of involving all levels of the organization (particularly those who do the work under review) in quality management, or wall-to-wall quality; the need to collect continuously aggregate data in lieu of "inspection" of individual cases; "doing it right the first time"; and listening to the customer. These familiar concepts, now embraced by hospitals, have profoundly affected how the JCAHO measures the quality of the hospital programs it surveys and accredits.

As previously stated, for many years the JCAHO emphasized the quality assurance program as a separate function or department, responsible for the annual review and reapproval of a quality assurance plan. Hospital departments also were expected to develop quality assurance plans that could be produced for surveyors or other interested parties. The medical staff was expected to participate in various quality assurance activities under the "peer review" umbrella. These plans and functions, in the absence of any glaring problems, were considered to be evidence of the hospital's high-quality care. This structural approach to quality management emphasized the institution's capability to provide high-quality care; it did not require proof to that effect.

In 1984 the JCAHO shifted its emphasis from structural requirements in quality assurance to the process of assuring quality or, more correctly, to quality review. The phrase "monitoring and evaluation," emphasizing as it does the notion of ongoing activity, became the key to "a program of systematic review that is integrated and coordinated and that results in the resolution of problems and the successful pursuit of opportunities to improve care," in the words of the president of the JCAHO, Dennis O'Leary, M.D.[10] Quality assurance committees and their staffs were instructed in the need for ongoing monitoring of clinical activities, the aggregation of monitoring data into information on trends, and the need to analyze, disseminate, and act on the knowledge gained from this process. Much of this shift occurred simultaneously with the first hospital experiences with Medicare's prospective payment system and the growing realization that hospitals were operating under new rules and were, therefore, in need of new management approaches in this more competitive environment.

Hospitals and the JCAHO realized that quality in health care, as in industry, cannot be applied to the product but must be an organic component of the process. As quality increasingly was recognized as the single most important preoccupation of the organization, managers saw the need for commitment to quality to extend throughout the depth and breadth of the organization. Just as the Ford Motor Company declared that "Quality Is Job One," hospitals adapted similar philosophies as they embraced top-quality care as the best competitive position. The evolution from structurally oriented, committee-driven quality assurance to organizationwide quality improvement grew from a better understanding within the organization of the meaning and importance of quality and from external forces that continued to demand more accountability and efficiency in the provision of care.[11]

With the introduction of its "Agenda for Change" in 1986, the Joint Commission on Accreditation of Healthcare Organizations announced two new goals: to improve the JCAHO's ability to evaluate health care organizations and to foster greater concern for the quality of patient care. Underlying concepts of the agenda are as follows:

- Patient outcomes are influenced by all activities of a healthcare organization. Effectiveness and efficiency in meeting the needs of patients results from the combined efforts of trustees, management, patient care professionals, and the support services of the organization.
- Continuous improvement in the quality of care provided to patients should be a priority of the healthcare organization.
- The focus of the Joint Commission should be on those activities of the healthcare organization that have the most significant impact on quality of care.
- The traditional Joint Commission focus on compliance with standards should be supplemented by collection, analysis, and feedback of data that reflect actual performance in key activities.[12]

The agenda included standards redirection, a reduction in the number and complexity of standards, a new focus on key functions, and an emphasis of standards that provide a foundation for continual improvement. Sets of clinical indicators were to be developed, and a centralized data base for the aggregation of clinical performance data developed under JCAHO auspices. Finally, the agenda discussed the need for a revised corporate culture within hospitals to support the new emphasis on the organization's performance in providing high-quality care.[13] The clinical indicators for a range of several hospital services are expected to be in use by 1992 and will provide a standard set of key indicators for quality of care in U.S. hospitals.

The body of hospital management literature is pointing the way toward quality management issues, which will eventually find their way into standards. The prudent executive who anticipates this evolutionary process has the opportunity to put into place a system that will bring total quality management and continuous quality improvement concepts into the hospital organization *now*. Borrowed from Japanese management via American manufacturing and service industries, these concepts require some adaptation to health care organizations but promise to be effective approaches to the systems problems that plague all hospitals and frequently are the source of increased costs and deficient quality.

There is some disagreement about whether total quality management (TQM) represents cost savings to hospitals or actually increases costs through adding another layer to hospital bureaucracy and by calling old cost-saving techniques "total quality management."[14] However, most proponents believe that TQM represents an effective approach not only in dealing with quality improvement, but also in decreasing the costs of providing care by addressing hospitals' systems problems.

In its emphasis on "continuous and relentless improvement in the total process that provides care, not simply in the improved actions of individual professionals,"[15] TQM is seen as differing from the traditional quality assurance approach. The challenge in implementing TQM in a hospital setting is that its very values often conflict with the hierarchical and professionally dominated hospital culture. Total quality management challenges the status quo in its demand that the customer's needs drive the changes in the organization, that top management respond immediately to suggestions for change that come from hospital staff (rather than "studying" the suggestions until they are no longer relevant), and that problems in health care organizations generally stem not from staff or people errors but from "the inability of the structure — within which all personnel function — to perform adequately."[16]

In implementing TQM in hospitals, a key issue is the conflict between professional authority and two direct results of TQM: constant inquiry and constant escalation of standards. Professionals typically seek a generally accepted community standard against which to measure themselves and their colleagues' performance. Inherent in TQM is the notion that once a standard of performance is met a new, higher standard must be set and achieved.

A further conflict arises for a hospital's traditional problem-solving hierarchy (doctors deal with doctors' problems, nurses deal with nurses' problems, and so forth). In TQM, problem-solving teams are oriented toward functions that cut across professions and are thus multidisciplinary; because the process focuses on the system, all disciplines must collaborate on the solution. Success depends on a certain amount of "leveling" taking place within the team, and traditional roles may be difficult to shed.

Another departure from traditional approaches to managing quality is the explicit recognition of attributes of the competition required by TQM. Not only is the competition recognized, but its best qualities are measured so that its product can be surpassed. This process, known as *benchmarking,* also recognizes that the customer's experience is the yardstick against which the competition is measured and implies that the goal the organization strives to meet is fluid and like the search for quality, will escalate constantly.[17]

McLaughlin and Kaluzny[18] identify 11 actions necessary for the successful implementation of TQM in the hospital setting:

1. Redefine the role of the professional to include the ability to be flexible and to strive for continuous improvement.
2. Redefine the corporate culture to avoid the "quick fix" in favor of the steady, continuous quest for quality.
3. Redefine the role of management so that frontline managers lead the process of change and top management allocates resources and

   manages the culture, leaving decision making to lower levels of
   management.
   4. Empower the staff to analyze and solve problems.
   5. Change organizational objectives so that programs set their own
      quality objectives, which evolve over time.
   6. Develop mentoring capacity to support risk taking at all levels of
      the organization.
   7. Drive the benchmarking process from the top; that is, top manage-
      ment has the ability to assess the environment and measure the
      competition.
   8. Modify the reward system to reward both performance and process
      development; as much as possible, confer nonfinancial rewards, such
      as continuing education programs.
   9. Look outside the health care industry for models of consumer-
      driven quality.
  10. Set realistic time frames for adopting and internalizing TQM; three
      to five years is standard.
  11. Make the TQM program a model for continuous improvement
      throughout the entire organization.

An institutionwide commitment to a process of continuous quality
improvement will position the hospital to make immediate use of new technology and new approaches to providing the highest quality of care. A further benefit of TQM is the knowledge that compliance with the JCAHO's
standards is virtually assured. Clinical indicators not already in use easily
can be integrated into such a process, relying as it does on ongoing data
collection, analysis, and action.
   Although the direction the JCAHO will take cannot be predicted, certain conclusions are clear:

  • Competition among health care organizations will only increase.
  • Consumers will continue to demand cost controls and better quality.
  • Quality requirements will continue to drive organizational planning
    and resource allocation.
  • Quality management is not a separate function within the organiza-
    tion; it must be the primary driving impulse behind the activities of
    each person in the organization.

   The development and refinement of quality indicators must be an ongoing task. There is considerable debate not only on the measurement of quality
but also on its relationship to variables and the question of who should
be responsible for quality measurement (physicians have a significant investment in the outcome of the process). In designing a quality-monitoring

process for a cardiovascular program, the following should be considered as starting points:

- Percentage of normal cardiac catheterizations
- Death rates for all procedures
- Percentage of emergency procedures
- Percentage of PTCAs that go to emergency surgery
- Catheters used per case
- Procedure time for all cases
- Cross-clamp time
- Percentage of procedures that need to be redone
- Use of blood and blood products from blood bank

Cardiac quality indicators will vary with place and time. Differences in length of stay, type of procedures, complication rates, and other indicators will be compared among institutions, cities, and regions. The process of identifying and adopting these indicators must allow for the widest possible representation of the medical staff. At the same time, care needs to be taken to ensure that the indicators do not become so diluted as to be ineffective in screening for quality problems. Quality management will become more aggressive in the future as the quality imperative becomes stronger and the costs associated with failure in this process become more evident. Having in place a system of indicators will allow the program to become more aggressive as the external environment dictates and as the internal environment requires.

Summary

Management involves focusing an organization's efforts toward the accomplishment of stated goals and objectives. In the context of a cardiovascular program, discrete management functions essential to the organization's success include planning and setting objectives, making decisions, organizing, staffing, directing, and exerting control. Decision making is the principal *task* of management. Decisions require objectives that are clearly stated and access to data from which to derive the information necessary to make decisions. Cardiovascular management information needs were presented and outlines for action recommended. Leadership, the most important *function* of management, was presented as it relates to the medical staff. Product line management and its application to an effective cardiovascular services program were discussed. A planning tool for cardiovascular product line development—a product line inventory—was examined, along with a sample showing general services and product line services in seven categories. Medical direction, program linkage, and joint ventures were explored as management options. Structuring a dedicated catheterization laboratory applying management principles; delegating responsibility; selecting and allocating properly trained staff (catheterization laboratory and cardiovascular surgery); and managing information in a developing or new CV program were detailed. Finally, quality management was reviewed as an emerging strategic imperative.

☐ *References*

1. Webber, J. B., and Peters, J. P. *Strategic Thinking: New Frontier for Hospital Management.* Chicago: American Hospital Publishing, 1983 [out of print].

2. Gardner, J. *On Leadership.* New York City: The Free Press, 1990, pp. 11–22.

3. Filley, A. C. *Interpersonal Conflict Resolution.* Glenview, IL: Scott, Foresman and Company, 1975.

4. Massie, J. L. *Essentials of Management.* Englewood Cliffs, NJ: Prentice-Hall, 1971, pp. 87–88.

5. The Flexner Report was compiled by the Carnegie Foundation for the Advancement of Teaching at the request of the American Medical Association. It examined the state of American medical schools in the first decade of this century and exposed the frequently poor quality of medical education in the United States. For a detailed description of the report and its historical context, see *The Social Transformation of American Medicine,* by Paul Starr (New York City: Basic Books, 1982).

6. Deming, W. E. *Out of Crisis.* Cambridge, MA: MIT Press, 1986.

7. Juran, J. *Management Breakthrough.* New York City: McGraw-Hill, 1964.

8. Crosby, P. *Quality Is Free.* New York City: Mentor Books, 1979.

9. *Quality Assurance in Home Care and Hospice Organizations.* Oakbrook Terrace, IL: Joint Commission on Accreditation of Healthcare Organizations, 1990.

10. *Accreditation Manual for Hospitals.* Chicago: Joint Commission on Accreditation of Hospitals, 1985, foreword.

11. *Committed to Quality.* Oakbrook Terrace, IL: Joint Commission on Accreditation of Healthcare Organizations, 1990.

12. *Quality Assurance in Home Care and Hospice Organizations.* Oakbrook Terrace, IL: Joint Commission on Accreditation of Healthcare Organizations, 1990.

13. *Committed to Quality.* Oakbrook Terrace, IL: Joint Commission on Accreditation of Healthcare Organizations, 1990.

14. Burda, D. Total quality management becomes big business. *Modern Healthcare* 21(4):25–29, Jan. 28, 1991.

15. McLaughlin, C. P., and Kaluzny, A. D. Total quality management in health: making it work. *Health Care Management Review* 15(3):7–14, Summer 1990.

16. McLaughlin and Kaluzny.

17. McLaughlin and Kaluzny.

18. McLaughlin and Kaluzny.

Chapter 6

Financial Management

Certain aspects of financial management are of particular interest to managers and directors of cardiovascular services. Whether one is assessing the feasibility of adding a new service, expanding a current service, or evaluating the performance of an existing one, key issues must be addressed. This chapter discusses five key issues:

1. Assessing feasibility and financial performance (including a brief overview of financial terminology and principles and revenue and cost management)
2. Reimbursement issues and future patterns of reimbursement
3. Pricing
4. Coding
5. Financial management for cardiovascular services

A financial model is presented that will help managers formulate, develop, and implement a long-term financial management strategy for a new, expanded, or revised CV program.

Assessing Feasibility and Financial Performance

Essentially two major functions are performed in the financial management process that require development of complex financial models. The first involves assessment of the financial feasibility of developing a new service or significantly changing existing services. The second uses financial models in evaluating and analyzing the financial performance of a set of interrelated services. This section outlines the process of assessing feasibility and financial performance. A generic cardiovascular services financial model will be presented and discussed. On the basis of certain assumptions (income, cash flow, distributions, return on investment, and such), a working computer model has been set up in tables 6-1 through 6-4 (pp. 132–39).

Financial Feasibility

The term *feasibility* connotes profitability. A *feasibility assessment,* therefore, evaluates the resources needed for a given course of action and predicts the financial outcome (profitability) of the project over a specified period of time. These predictions are based on a set of interlocking assumptions about the product or service being considered: demand for it, market share captured, prices charged for it, and expenses generated to produce a given level or volume of that product or service.

A financial feasibility assessment is necessary for the development of a new cardiac catheterization service or the development of a cardiovascular surgery service. In either of these cases, a market assessment is performed to calculate total demand for cardiac catheterization and/or cardiovascular surgery and interventional cardiology procedures. Assumptions are then formulated about the market share the program could capture for these services. (These methodologies were discussed in chapter 3.)

Next, a description of the program is prepared, outlining the modifications needed at the facility that will provide the new program; the equipment, architectural services, and staff training; and other costs that will be incurred during program development. These expenses represent the capital investment required for initiating the program or service.

Assumptions are then made regarding the pricing for individual products or services that will be made available through the program. These products and services may include cardiac catheterization on both an inpatient and outpatient basis, various cardiovascular surgery procedures, and interventional cardiology procedures such as percutaneous transluminal coronary angioplasty (PTCA). More and more the pricing of hospital services is based on fixed case price reimbursement, such as that provided for under Medicare's current prospective payment system, where each diagnosis-related group (DRG) provides for a relatively fixed level of reimbursement.

The most complex part of the feasibility assessment is developing expense assumptions. A variety of expenses — direct and indirect, fixed and variable, and capital costs — are associated with a project of this nature. Obviously, the degree to which these assumptions can be refined and accurately predicted will affect the value of the model and, ultimately, the projected financial statements drawn from the model.

Proper determination of expense assumptions involves a variety of individuals, including physicians and staff members who have experience with the service being developed. Because information gathered from other programs is extremely helpful, the feasibility assessment process can benefit from the use of outside consultants.

Certain historical data can be especially useful to a financial feasibility study—for example, a record of patients who entered the planning hospital (or its medical staff practice) but were referred out because the hospital lacked the appropriate service. In the case of cardiac catheterization feasibility assessment, knowing the number of patients who were admitted but then transferred to another hospital because catheterization was unavailable helps project the actual number of cardiac catheterizations that could be generated by the planning hospital. However, this is not a reliable source for these patient data, because many patients never enter that hospital in the first place, knowing these services do not exist there. A hospital considering the addition of cardiovascular surgery to its invasive diagnostic program will find a detailed record of the disposition of all cases essential. Such a record includes not only cases deemed normal but also those referred out for interventional procedures—including PTCA and cardiovascular surgery.

These data result in a *yield rate of cardiac cases,* which can predict actual volumes that can be controlled within a given market area by the proposed CV program. This number is used to verify demand and market share projections that are made during the market assessment process. However, total demand for the new procedures cannot be completely explained by using the yield rate based on current utilization because, once again, many cases may not be referred to a diagnostic-only catheterization laboratory where no interventional cardiology procedures are performed or where no cardiovascular surgery backup is available. Referring physicians frequently prefer to refer their cases to cardiologists who work at full-service cardiovascular facilities.

During feasibility assessment for cardiovascular surgery and interventional cardiology, the number of diagnostic catheterizations will increase. To compensate, it is necessary to reduce the total number of diagnostic cardiac catheterizations included in the model to "net out" the current volume so that interim diagnostic catheterizations are recorded.

Spin-off revenue is possible from the addition of a cardiovascular service, and this should be taken into account when determining feasibility. Spin-off revenue is the direct result of the added cardiovascular patients and their consumption of cardiac and noncardiac services; more important, the addition allows the hospital and its medical staff to access consumers who have noncardiac conditions that require treatment or who present with cardiac disease as a comorbid condition. For example, a patient who needs a cholecystectomy and has a cardiac condition typically will be referred by the attending physician to a surgeon who can perform the procedure in a hospital that also has cardiovascular surgery, which might be needed for backup. By adding cardiovascular surgery, a hospital also can *recapture* patients, which will significantly enhance overall volume.

Table 6-1. Computer Model: Basic Assumptions

3-NOV-90   WK3   BASIC ASSUMPTIONS

UTILIZATION ASSUMPTIONS

		Year 1	Year 2	Year 3	Year 4	Year 5	Year 6	Year 7	Year 8	Year 9	Year 10
Cardiovascular Surgery			150	175	200	225	250	275	300	300	300
	Ratio to CVS										
Catheterization	500%		750	875	1000	1125	1250	1375	1500	1500	1500
PTCA	100%		150	175	200	225	250	275	300	300	300
Vascular Surgery	50%		75	88	100	113	125	138	150	150	150
Total		0	1125	1313	1500	1688	1875	2063	2250	2250	2250

PRICING ASSUMPTIONS

CVS	$28,000	Cath-In	$4,000
PTCA	$9,000	Cath-Out	$2,500
		Vasc.	$15,000

INFLATION ASSUMPTIONS

(Rates begin in 1993; compounded thereafter)

Revenue	8%
Salaries	8%
Supplies	5%
Utilities	6%

REVENUE ADJUSTMENTS

Bad Debt	10%
Contractual Allow	20%

STAFFING ASSUMPTIONS

	Fixed Hrs./Week	Variable Hrs./Unit	Hourly Wage
Management	80	0.0	$25.14
Radiology Tech. (PTCA)	10	4.0	$11.74
Cath Lab Nurses (PTCA)	20	8.0	$16.06
C.V. Tech. (PTCA)	10	4.0	$14.03
DX Cath Team	N/A	6.0	$12.66
O.R. Supervisor	40	0.0	$17.10

EXPENSE ASSUMPTIONS

	FIXED COSTS	VARIABLE COSTS PER MONTH	
Category	Per Month	Var. Rate	Variable Unit
Medical Director	$10,000		
Perfusion		$1,000	Per CVS
Employee Benefits		18%	Salaries & Wages
Marketing	$10,000		
Legal & Accounting	$500		
Laundry and Central Supply			
Insurance			
Medical Supplies (CVS)		$300	Per CVS
Pharmacy Supplies (CVS)		$250	Per CVS
PTCA Supplies (Incl. Pharm.)		$3,500	Per CVS
DX Cath Supplies		$1,600	Per CVS
Med/Surg supplies		$1,400	Per PTCA
CSICU Supplies		$400	Per Cath
Vasc. Surg. Costs		$100	Per Inpatient Day
Admin. Supplies		$150	Per Inpatient Day
		35%	Gross Charges
		$5	Per Procedure

O.R. Nurses	30	12.0	$15.16	
O.R. Support	10	5.0	$8.35	
CSICU Supervisor	40	0.0	$21.70	
Clerical	80	2.0	$8.17	
Nursing Hours / Critical Care Day		22.0	$16.46	
Hospital Manhours / Patient Day		30.0	$14.00	
Stand-by & Call Back/Mo.	$12,000			

AVG LENGTH OF STAY	CSICU	MED-SURG
PTCA	1.0	3.0
CVS	3.0	8.0
Inpatient Cath	0.0	2.5

Inpatient/Outpatient Assumptions

Outpatient Cath Rate	75.0%
Caths in DRGs 104 and 106	12.5%

	Value	Rate	Basis
Utilities	$150	$0	Per Square Foot
Printing	$150	$5	Per Procedure
Telephone		$6	Per Procedure
Minor Equipment	$2,500	$150	Per Cardiac Surgery
Repairs & Maintenance			
Dues & Subscriptions	$250	0.67%	Equip. Purchase Price
Travel	$1,500		
Depreciation--			
Building	$10,712		
Equipment	$110,000		
Office Furnishings	$0		
Amortization	$2,083		
Miscellaneous		2%	Net Revenue

Table 6-2. Computer Model: Capital Cost Assumptions

3-NOV-90   WK3   CAPITAL COST ASSUMPTIONS

EQUIPMENT COST ASSUMPTIONS

Laboratory	$75,000
Operating Room	2,500,000
Anesthesia	75,000
Respiratory Care	75,000
CSICU	1,000,000
Catheterization Laboratory	2,000,000
Cardiac Rehabilitation	800,000
Expense contingency 7%	$20,000
Total	$6,600,000

CONSTRUCTION COST ASSUMPTIONS

Total Square Footage	8,000
Construction Costs per Square Foot	$260
Architect & Engineering, Fees & Permits	18%
Contingency	10%
Equipment Lease	$0
Total Construction Costs	$2,080,000
Add'l Mech. & Elec. Upgrades	331,500
Architect & Engineering, Fees & Permits	434,070
Contingency	284,557
Total Construction Budget	$3,130,127

OTHER CAPITAL ASSUMPTIONS

Construction Period (Months)	8
Construction Draw Rate	50.0%
Equipment Useful Life for Depr (Years)	5
Building Depreciable Life (Years)	25.0
Start-up Costs	$250,000
Start-up Costs Amortization Life (Years)	10

DEBT SERVICE COMPUTATIONS

Note Total	$10,063,597
Interest Rate	8.0%
Term (Years)	10

CAPITAL EXPENDED

Land	$0
Major Equipment	6,600,000
Construction	3,130,127
Start-up Costs	250,000
Office Furnishings	0
Capitalized Interest	83,470
Total	$10,063,597

OTHER CASH ASSUMPTIONS

Days in Accts Receivable	
Days in Accts Payable	
Cash Reserves	
% of Monthly Operating Expenses in Other Liabilities	
Inventory	

Principal & Interest Payments

	1992	1993	1994	1995	1996	1997	1998	1999
Interest	$0	$780,338	$723,496	$661,935	$595,265	$523,062	$444,866	$360,180
Principal Payments	0	684,852	741,695	803,255	869,925	942,128	1,020,324	1,105,011
Total Payments	$0	$1,465,190	$1,465,190	$1,465,190	$1,465,190	$1,465,190	$1,465,190	$1,465,190

Table 6-3. Computer Model: Income Statement

3-NOV-90   WK3   INCOME STATEMENT

	Year 1	Year 2	Year 3	Year 4	Year 5	Year 6	Year 7	Year 8	Year 9	Year 10
REVENUES										
Cardiovascular Surgery	$0	$4,536,000	$5,715,360	$7,054,387	$8,571,080	$10,285,297	$12,218,932	$14,396,124	$15,547,814	$16,791,639
Catheterization	0	1,923,750	2,423,925	2,991,816	3,635,056	4,362,068	5,182,136	6,105,499	6,593,939	7,121,454
PTCA	0	1,458,000	1,837,080	2,267,482	2,754,990	3,305,988	3,927,514	4,627,326	4,997,512	5,397,312
Vascular Surgery	0	1,215,000	1,530,900	1,889,568	2,295,825	2,754,990	3,272,928	3,856,105	4,164,593	4,497,760
Gross Revenues	0	9,132,750	11,507,265	14,203,253	17,256,952	20,708,343	24,601,511	28,985,053	31,303,857	33,808,166
Revenue Deductions										
Bad Debts	0	(913,275)	(1,150,727)	(1,420,325)	(1,725,695)	(2,070,834)	(2,460,151)	(2,898,505)	(3,130,386)	(3,380,817)
Contractual Disallowances	0	(1,826,550)	(2,301,453)	(2,840,651)	(3,451,390)	(4,141,669)	(4,920,302)	(5,797,011)	(6,260,771)	(6,761,633)
Total Revenue Deductions	0	(2,739,825)	(3,452,180)	(4,260,976)	(5,177,086)	(6,212,503)	(7,380,453)	(8,695,516)	(9,391,157)	(10,142,450)
Net Revenues	0	6,392,925	8,055,086	9,942,277	12,079,867	14,495,840	17,221,058	20,289,537	21,912,700	23,665,716
OPERATING EXPENSES										
S&W -- Management	0	112,949	121,985	131,744	142,283	153,666	165,959	179,236	193,575	209,061
S&W -- Rad Tech	0	14,201	16,706	19,522	22,680	26,220	30,180	34,607	37,375	40,366
S&W -- Cath Lab Nurses	0	38,852	45,707	53,410	62,052	71,736	82,572	94,683	102,257	110,438
S&W -- C.V. Tech	0	16,971	19,965	23,329	27,104	31,334	36,067	41,357	44,666	48,239
S&W -- DX Cath Team	0	61,528	77,525	95,688	116,261	139,513	165,741	195,273	210,895	227,767
S&W -- OR Supervisor	0	38,413	41,487	44,805	48,390	52,261	56,442	60,957	65,834	71,101
S&W -- OR Nurses	0	55,013	64,718	75,625	87,863	101,574	116,917	134,065	144,790	156,373
S&W -- OR Support	0	11,453	13,587	15,988	18,687	21,716	25,110	28,907	31,220	33,717
S&W -- Clerical	0	56,559	64,658	73,690	83,753	94,955	107,413	121,257	130,957	141,434
S&W -- CSICU	0	283,401	348,310	421,792	504,801	598,393	703,728	822,087	887,854	958,883
S&W -- Other	0	1,010,273	1,244,950	1,510,710	1,811,023	2,149,719	2,531,015	2,959,560	3,196,325	3,452,031
Employee Benefits	0	305,930	370,727	443,934	526,482	619,396	723,806	840,958	908,235	980,894
Medical Director	0	129,600	139,968	151,165	163,259	176,319	190,425	205,659	222,112	239,881
Perfusion	0	162,000	204,120	251,942	306,110	367,332	436,390	514,147	555,279	599,701
Marketing	0	126,000	132,300	138,915	145,861	153,154	160,811	168,852	177,295	186,159
Legal & Accounting	0	6,300	6,615	6,946	7,293	7,658	8,041	8,443	8,865	9,308

Laundry	0	47,250	57,881	69,458	82,047	95,721	110,558	126,639	132,971	139,620
Insurance	0	39,375	48,234	57,881	68,372	92,341	101,575	110,809	110,809	116,350
Medical Supplies	0	551,250	675,281	810,338	957,211	1,116,746	1,289,842	1,477,455	1,551,328	1,628,895
Pharmacy Supplies	0	252,000	308,700	370,440	437,582	510,513	589,642	675,408	709,179	744,638
Inpatient Supplies	0	15,750	21,278	23,153	27,349	31,907	36,853	42,213	44,324	46,540
PTCA and Cath Supplies	0	535,500	655,988	787,185	929,862	1,084,839	1,252,989	1,435,242	1,507,005	1,582,355
Vascular Surgery Costs	0	425,250	535,815	661,349	803,539	964,247	1,145,525	1,349,637	1,457,608	1,574,216
Admin. Supplies	0	9,056	10,543	12,155	13,902	15,794	17,840	20,051	21,054	22,106
Utilities	0	30,528	32,360	34,301	36,359	38,541	40,853	43,305	45,903	48,657
Printing	0	7,796	9,220	10,766	12,444	14,262	16,232	18,363	19,281	20,245
Telephone	0	8,978	10,667	12,502	14,495	16,655	18,996	21,529	22,605	23,735
Minor Equipment	0	31,500	33,075	34,729	63,814	71,791	80,406	89,703	99,728	110,532
Repairs & Maintenance	0	554,400	582,120	611,226	641,787	673,877	707,570	742,949	780,096	819,101
Dues & Subscriptions	0	3,150	3,308	3,473	3,647	3,829	4,020	4,221	4,432	4,654
Travel	0	18,900	19,845	20,837	21,879	22,973	24,122	25,328	26,594	27,924
Interest	0	780,338	723,496	661,935	595,265	523,062	444,866	360,180	268,464	169,136
Depreciation and Amortization	0	1,473,544	1,473,544	1,473,544	1,473,544	1,473,544	153,544	153,544	153,544	153,544
Miscellaneous	0	127,859	161,102	198,846	241,597	289,917	344,421	405,791	438,254	473,314
Total Expenses	0	7,341,865	8,275,782	9,313,322	10,498,599	11,805,504	11,920,473	13,512,414	14,310,712	15,170,913
NET INCOME (LOSS)	$0	($948,940)	($220,697)	$628,955	$1,581,267	$2,690,336	$5,300,585	$6,777,123	$7,601,988	$8,494,803

Table 6-4. Computer Model: Cash Flow, Distributions, and Return on Investment

3-NOV-90   WK3   CASH FLOW, DISTRIBUTIONS, AND RETURN ON INVESTMENT

	Year 1	Year 2	Year 3	Year 4	Year 5	Year 6	Year 7	Year 8	Year 9	Year 10
SOURCES OF CASH										
Net Income (Loss)	$0	($948,940)	($220,697)	$628,955	$1,581,267	$2,690,336	$5,300,585	$6,777,123	$7,601,988	$8,494,803
Add: Deprec. and Amort.	0	1,473,544	1,473,544	1,473,544	1,473,544	1,473,544	153,544	153,544	153,544	153,544
Cash from Operations	0	524,604	1,252,847	2,102,499	3,054,811	4,163,880	5,454,129	6,930,667	7,755,532	8,648,347
Increase in Accounts Payable	0	380,027	69,778	76,338	87,633	94,932	102,168	112,023	55,353	59,574
Increase in Other Liabilities	0	42,828	5,448	6,052	6,914	7,624	671	9,286	4,657	5,018
Issuance of Debt	0	10,063,597	0	0	0	0	0	0	0	0
Equity Investment	0	1,208,435	0	0	0	0	0	0	0	0
Total Sources of Cash	0	12,219,490	1,328,073	2,184,890	3,149,359	4,266,436	5,556,968	7,051,976	7,815,542	8,712,939
USES OF CASH										
Capital Expenditures	0	9,813,597	0	0	0	0	0	0	0	0
Principal Payments on Debt	0	684,852	741,695	803,255	869,925	942,128	1,020,324	1,105,011	1,196,726	1,296,054
Increase in Accts Receivable	0	1,226,040	318,771	361,927	409,949	463,337	522,645	588,475	311,292	336,195
Increase in Inventory	0	225,000	0	0	0	0	0	0	0	0
Start-up Costs	0	250,000	0	0	0	0	0	0	0	0
Total Uses of Cash	0	12,199,490	1,060,465	1,165,182	1,279,874	1,405,466	1,542,969	1,693,486	1,508,018	1,632,249
Net Cash Flow	0	20,000	267,608	1,019,707	1,869,485	2,860,970	4,013,999	5,358,490	6,307,524	7,080,690
Beginning Cash Balance	0	0	20,000	287,608	1,307,315	3,176,800	6,037,771	10,051,769	15,410,259	21,717,783
Cash Before Distributions	0	20,000	287,608	1,307,315	3,176,800	6,037,771	10,051,769	15,410,259	21,717,783	28,798,473
Cash Distributions	0	0	0	0	0	0	0	0	0	0
Ending Cash Balance	$0	$20,000	$287,608	$1,307,315	$3,176,800	$6,037,771	$10,051,769	$15,410,259	$21,717,783	$28,798,473

Financial Return Calculations for Six-Year Investment Period

Initial Invested Capital $1,208,435

Hurdle Interest Rate   10.0%

Internal Rate of Return   69.4%

Net Present Value $12,556,566

There is no question that by adding a cardiac catheterization program or cardiovascular surgery to its diagnostic program a hospital will increase its volume of noninvasive cardiac tests. However, the volume of these procedures can be neither predicted accurately nor included in the financial projections owing to the different ownership of these services.

The principal component of feasibility is *financial* in nature. An assessment, however, should also address operational, political, and strategic feasibility.

Operational Feasibility

The assessment of operational feasibility helps determine whether a facility can handle the addition of complex services such as cardiovascular surgery and interventional cardiology. Projections must consider what the addition of surgical procedures will mean in terms of expanded operations—postoperative recovery of patients and the consequent demand for critical care and monitored beds, for example. The results of an operational feasibility assessment can significantly affect the project's financial feasibility as operational feasibility is turned into capital requirement assumptions. Finally, the issue of capability extends to the medical staff, the clinical staff, and the management staff in their respective abilities to handle expanded operations.

Political Feasibility

Political feasibility gauges the willingness of the medical staff or the community at large to support a certain addition—for example, a catheterization laboratory without cardiovascular surgery or cardiovascular surgery at relatively low volumes. Although market statistics, as well as the hospital's historical market penetration, might suggest that a sufficient number of patients can be captured to make the program profitable, this may be misleading. If the medical community resists the program on political grounds, desired market share will not be attained, patients will not support the program, physicians will not refer patients (at least not in the volume needed), and therefore the program will not be feasible.

Strategic Feasibility

Strategic feasibility relates to the ability to implement a clinical program successfully in a competitive environment. Strategic factors, such as competitive action or reaction, certificate-of-need legislation, managed care contracts, and so on, may preclude an otherwise successful program from achieving sufficient volume or from being implemented at all due to licensing restrictions. All of these factors affect the overall feasibility assessment.

Financial Feasibility Model

A financial model can be used not only to determine the financial feasibility of a planned project or program but also to evaluate the future of an existing one.

A financial model is a computer program that generates financial projections of a project (or a department or an enterprise). The projections may cover one or more periods (months, quarters, or years). To generate the financial projections, the person using the model must make numerous assumptions. With a catheterization laboratory used as an example, some of the assumptions that must be made include:

- Number of inpatient and outpatient diagnostic cardiac catheterizations
- Pricing for inpatient and outpatient catheterizations
- Personnel required
- Salaries
- Supply costs per procedure
- Equipment required
- Source of required funds

Each of these assumptions must be made for each projection period.

The computer can be programmed to process all these assumptions very quickly to produce the financial projections. After reviewing the projections, the user may determine that some assumptions need to be changed to portray the expected operations more accurately.

In addition, the user may want to experiment with "what if" scenarios by changing one or more assumptions to see what effect the change has on the financial projections. For example, a user may want to determine the effect on net income (the "bottom line") of increasing the price for inpatient diagnostic cardiac catheterizations by 10 percent a year beginning in year 2 of the projection period.

The model in tables 6-1 through 6-4 shows the type of assumptions needed and the resulting financial reports. (Note: The numbers in the financial projections are for illustrative purposes only and under no circumstances should be used as a guide in making assumptions for a cardiovascular services feasibility assessment.)

Table 6-1 summarizes basic assumptions for the program:

- Utilization
- Pricing
- Revenue adjustments
- Staffing (fixed and variable)
- Average length of stay

- Inflation
- Expenses (fixed and variable)

Table 6-2 summarizes capital cost assumptions:

- Equipment costs
- Construction costs
- Construction period
- Depreciable lives
- Start-up costs
- Days in accounts receivable
- Days in accounts payable
- Cash reserves
- Inventory
- Debt and equity

Table 6-3 is a detailed projected income statement for all of the projection periods.

Table 6-4 is a cash flow, distributions, and return on investment statement for all of the projection periods. At the end of this statement are the following summary items:

- *Initial invested capital:* The total cash required for the project, minus debt incurred (if any).
- *Hurdle interest rate:* The minimum rate of return required by a hospital, in this example 10 percent.
- *Internal rate of return (IRR):* That discount rate that equates the present value of a project's expected cash inflows to the present value of the project's expected costs. Thus, the IRR of a project would be 0 percent if the net present value (NPV) of the project's cash inflows equaled the NPV of the project's cash outflows. An IRR greater than 0 percent indicates a positive NPV (that is, the NPV of the cash inflows is greater than the NPV of the project's cash outflows). The larger the IRR, the better the project is from a financial standpoint.
- *Net present value (NPV):* The discounted value of all cash inflows and all cash outflows of the project, assuming a particular discount rate. For many hospitals, this discount rate is the hurdle interest rate. The larger the NPV, the better the project is from a financial standpoint.

Measures of Financial Performance

The principal measure of financial performance is always profitability, the excess of revenues over expenses. This is the goal toward which all financial management aims. The central focus in the preceding model (and for any model that serves as a tool for financial analysis) is the profit and loss (or income) statement (see table 6-3).

Whereas the finance department can develop a program-specific income statement based on actual or estimated financial results, the program manager might not be able to tell which variables affect the revenues and expenses associated with program profitability. By developing a model similar to the one in tables 6-1 through 6-4, the manager is forced to concentrate on the assumptions that underlie the program. Consequently, it is possible to identify and trace the source of inefficiency, miscommunication, faulty assumptions, and other errors and omissions.

Used in this way, the financial model becomes a tool for ongoing analysis of the financial performance of the program. Analysis, however, is without value unless it leads to action.

Role of Physicians in Financial Performance or Feasibility

The principal determinant of case cost — and therefore financial feasibility or performance — is the quality of clinical practices among participating physicians. In projecting financial feasibility it is important to know the physicians who will provide patient care in the program under consideration; that is, the quality of financial performance will directly parallel the quality of physician practice patterns.

For cardiovascular surgery, detailed financial projections can be based on industry norms or community standards. Actual program performance, however, will center on the practice behavior of key players who may not even be identified or affiliated with the program yet: cardiovascular surgeons, cardiac anesthesiologists, intensivists, and other physicians. Therefore, although preliminary projections are necessary, they must be validated or adjusted in cooperation with the physicians who eventually join the program.

Financial Management: An Overview

Financial management can be summarized simply as those tasks that ensure the maximum financial performance for an organization. In large and complex organizations such as hospitals, these activities are increasingly the responsibility of specialists, for example, accountants, billers, collectors, coders, internal auditors, and controllers.

Although specialists will continue to perform functions crucial to the success of the hospital and the cardiovascular program, those directly involved in program management will play an equally important role in managing the financial performance. Program management's unique knowledge of day-to-

day operations must be combined with the specialists' expertise for effective management of the program's financial resources.

Cardiovascular program managers whose responsibility includes financial management of resources must know basic accounting principles and
have a grasp of financial reporting. Accordingly, it is recommended that
they receive training in fundamental accounting and financial management.
To provide a framework for the discussion on financial management, a brief
review of terminology and concepts follows.

Financial management basically is concerned with documenting *transactions*. These transactions, such as purchasing an electrode, paying a nurse,
or performing an electrocardiogram, form the foundation of all financial
management. All personnel and all computer equipment involved in financial management are intended to record, classify, and report these transactions efficiently so that financial reports are accurate and meaningful and
can be interpreted easily by program management.

Business transactions are mainly concerned with cash: A business spends
cash to purchase supplies and services and receives cash from the sale of
goods and services. To the extent that cash received exceeds cash spent, the
business is financially successful.

Although somewhat simplified as stated here, this description also
applies to cardiovascular program financial management, whose goal also
is *to spend less than is earned*. To understand transactions and how they
are recorded and analyzed, program managers should know these terms:

- *Expenses:* The supplies and services consumed in operating an enterprise. Expenses are of two kinds: fixed or variable. Fixed expenses
  remain the same each month, for example, a departmental manager's
  salary, membership dues, subscriptions, or utilities. Variable expenses
  fluctuate each month depending on the volume of department activity.
  Examples of variable expenses include medical supplies, pharmacy
  supplies, cine film, and laundry.
- *Direct expenses:* The expenses directly associated with a particular
  department; examples include supplies and wages.
- *Indirect expenses:* Also called *overhead expenses,* the expenses paid
  regularly but are not identified with a particular department; examples include electricity, insurance, and legal fees.
- *Cost accounting:* The process of analyzing direct and indirect costs as
  they relate to particular departments and specific services involving
  tracking (accounting for) expenses. Determining the cost of performing one EKG or the cost of one minute of surgery time is an example.
- *Capital expenditure:* The purchase of equipment whose life will exceed
  one year and whose cost will exceed a predetermined amount (for
  example, $50). Equipment with a life of less than one year and a cost
  that is less than the predetermined amount generally is deemed minor

equipment and is considered an expense for the period in which it is acquired.

- *Depreciation:* Charging the cost of a capital expenditure to a department over the estimated useful life of the equipment for accounting purposes. For example, if a hospital purchased a catheterization laboratory for $1,000,000 and estimated the equipment to have a useful life of 10 years, the hospital would record $100,000 each year as depreciation expense.
- *Classes of expenses:* Expenses categorized by type of expense. Examples include salaries, employee benefits, supplies, services, leases and rentals, and depreciation.
- *Accounts:* The records of expenses and revenues used to classify transactions involving particular items or exchanges. Each expense transaction is assigned to one account within a class of accounts. For example, catheters and copy machine paper both are supplies, but the former are medical supplies and the latter is part of office supplies. Each type of revenue transaction is also recorded in its own account.
- *Cost:* The amount paid for an expense or a capital expenditure. The terms *costs* and *expenses* are often used interchangeably.
- *Cost center:* Generally a department or a subdepartment. Costs (or expenses) are charged to the cost center to which they apply. For example, medical supplies are charged to the catheterization laboratory's cost center or to the cardiac rehabilitation department's cost center, depending on where the supplies were used.
- *Revenue:* Charges made to inpatients and outpatients for services performed or supplies provided to them that generate income (revenue).
- *Revenue deduction:* The difference between the hospital's full charges to patients and the amount actually collected. Because of service agreements with individual hospitals and providers, not all payers (Medicare, Medicaid, and managed care companies) pay full charges. In addition, individual patients sometimes fail to pay the bills for which they are responsible. Revenue deductions basically can be categorized as follows:
  - Contractual allowances (or contractual adjustments)
  - Bad debts (charges for patients who probably could pay but who for various reasons pay no part of their bills)
  - Charity (charges for patients who generally cannot pay any part of their bills)
  - Other (employees' discounts, courtesy discounts, and so forth)
- *Reimbursement:* Payment of the costs incurred in treating patients. Because of Medicare's history of paying for a hospital's costs rather than its charges, cost-based reimbursement was initiated. Whereas most business entities receive payment for services rendered, hospitals

continue to think in terms of receiving reimbursement for the costs
they incurred in treating an insured patient.

- *Profit and loss statement:* Also called a *statement of income, income statement,* or *P & L,* a periodic report that summarizes revenues and expenses for a certain period. When revenues minus revenue deductions exceeds expenses, a profit (or net income) results.
- *Balance sheet:* Statement that reports the hospital's assets (what it owns) and its liabilities (what it owes) at a particular point in time (generally the end of a month). The difference between the hospital's assets and liabilities is called its *equity* or *fund balance.*
- *Accounts receivable:* Charges to patients that remain unpaid.
- *Accounts payable:* Costs incurred (expenses and capital expenditures) that the hospital has not yet paid.

Managing Revenues

As noted earlier, financial management for a cardiovascular program must be premised on maximizing revenue while minimizing costs so as to achieve optimal profitability. In many respects, managing revenues has become much simpler under case-based revenue systems (such as Medicare's DRGs) and under the fixed price per diem systems used by managed care companies and, in some states, by Medicaid. These systems, which reimburse on the basis of a fixed sum per patient day, adjusted by type of bed used, all involve preestablished or negotiated rates, rather than relying strictly on the patient bill. In these arrangements, the type of procedure or length of stay determines the revenue rather than "à la carte" patient charges.

Managing revenue involves a combination of increasing patient volume and negotiating higher case rates and higher per diem rates with payers. Increasing patient volume is a function of marketing and is discussed later in this chapter and again in chapter 8.

Negotiating rates with managed care companies is a complex process requiring not only negotiation skills but also a firm knowledge of the market, the competition, and the payer. It also requires having a *strong* cardiovascular product. Although cardiovascular services have been the cornerstone of much managed care development, the high cost of care for patients with cardiac disease has made it necessary to approach patient services contracting from a *hospitalwide* perspective. This means that all the resources of the hospital's managed care and contracting personnel must be utilized.

Despite the trend toward cost-based revenue systems (and fixed price per diem systems), hospitals continue to generate patient bills that reflect all the services provided and supplies consumed during the patient's course of treatment, as recorded by the patient accounting system.

The *patient accounting system* accumulates units of services provided to individual patients and multiplies the number of units by the price found in the hospital's charge description master. The *charge description master* is a record of all goods (for example, catheters and pharmaceuticals) and services (CCU day, chest X ray, and so forth) the hospital provides, itemized by department and item price.

It is the responsibility of management to maintain item prices in accordance with local market conditions. The price of products and services generally also influences both sellers and buyers in consumer markets. The price of oil, for example, affects the price of gasoline, which ultimately affects the demand for, or amount of, gasoline consumed. However, hospital services are not generally price sensitive, principally because of the separation of the role of user (patient), selector (physician), and payer (insurance company or Medicare). Program management is responsible for maintaining individual item charges within an overall hospital pricing strategy or philosophy that can range from aggressive to conservative. Item prices should reflect both costs and market conditions. Conventional retail pricing reflects market conditions only, based on the reality that if costs exceed what the market will bear, the service should be eliminated. Regardless of the philosophy, regular management of prices is important.

Individual item prices are more important in outpatient services (such as cardiac rehabilitation or noninvasive cardiology) where competition exists. Prices charged by physicians' offices for similar services are an important source of competitive pricing information. Similar information for inpatient services, although more difficult to obtain, is an important source for evaluating pricing. When individual prices are not available, case prices, which are more accessible, are used. Because of managed care, case prices are the focus of competition for cardiovascular programs and other subspecialty services.

Managing Costs

Central to financial management is the control of costs, especially supply and personnel costs. These expenses have been difficult for hospitals to manage, because the medical staff itself determines how resources are consumed. Further, the number and variety of professionals involved in hospital operations makes cost control difficult to manage. For example, as patients are transported through a chain of departments, centralized control over the patient — and over the process — is lost. However, the trend toward program or service line management, rather than functional organization, is bringing new cost manageability to the health care industry.

For cardiovascular services, the move toward service line management is creating a more integrated, product-oriented approach to assessing costs.

Attention is placed on the resources consumed by a typical patient in a specific program for a specific procedure or with a specific DRG, rather than on evaluations of individual item costs or staffing levels in a particular unit. Case cost management, then, offers significant alternatives over supply price and staffing reductions. Other alternatives also must be considered, as discussed in the following sections.

Productivity

Productivity embodies the notion of decreasing inputs (supplies, services, or labor) while holding output constant or increasing output with a steady supply of input. This concept is most often applied to labor productivity but can be applied to all resource inputs.

Staffing

Labor, which generally exceeds 50 percent of all cardiovascular program costs, represents the single most significant resource expended in the delivery of cardiovascular services. Therefore, careful attention must be paid to staffing levels, staffing ratios, and personnel utilization.

Cross-Training

Improving labor productivity and enhancing staff skills frequently involve cross-training, which prepares individuals to perform multiple functions on a regular basis. Not only can cross-training increase production and reduce labor inputs, it can enhance employee morale.

Substitution

Substitution uses the least expensive resource (for example, less skilled personnel) to accomplish as many tasks as possible. Quality of performance, however, must be monitored regularly.

Supply Standardization

Standardizing supplies can cut costs, especially for high-volume, expensive items such as catheters or pacemakers. Even used conservatively, standardization can minimize costs associated with supply acquisition. For example, using multiple vendors not only can increase inventory cost, it can increase negotiation costs in terms of average unit price per item.

Inventory

Managing inventory is a function of the materials management personnel and cardiovascular services personnel. It is not uncommon for cardiac catheterization departments and cardiovascular operating rooms to overstock inventory. However, this practice increases inventory costs (longer stocking time, more time needed for record keeping, more insurance, more space requirements, and so forth). Therefore, it is incumbent on management personnel to hold inventory to a safe minimum.

Analysis of Per Unit Costs

A mechanism is needed to evaluate the per unit cost of performing certain procedures. This assists management personnel in evaluating the impact of fixed and variable costs on the delivery of services.

Procedure Times

The time it takes to perform various procedures can significantly affect overall program cost. Procedure times in the catheterization laboratory, for example, can vary considerably. Efforts to minimize procedure time as well as turnaround time between procedures can increase program profitability and marketability. Also, controlling procedure time makes scheduling easier and more accommodating for physicians.

Reimbursement Issues

Because of retrospective cost reimbursement under Medicare and Medicaid from 1966 through 1983, the term *reimbursement* is used to describe how hospitals generate revenue and receive cash. These programs reimbursed hospitals for their costs associated with providing care to insured patients. Blue Cross later adopted a modified cost-based approach to paying for hospital services. The following discussion reviews how particular programs pay for hospital services, with specific attention to applications unique to cardiovascular services.

Cardiovascular health care services can be divided into separate cost centers such as inpatient, outpatient, and physician services. To some extent these services overlap; for example, anesthesiologists sometimes are paid directly by the hospital and therefore are billed for under the inpatient hospital billing system. Physicians' offices often provide outpatient diagnostic procedures, and certain procedures are performed on both an inpatient and outpatient basis. This is true for noninvasive diagnostic tests and, with increasing frequency, for diagnostic cardiac catheterization. Bills from providers historically were submitted to various payers on the basis of their organizational affiliations. As such, hospitals submitted bills for their services associated with an incident or course of treatment. Inpatient services were aggregated and submitted on one bill for one course of treatment or length of stay. Outpatient services were submitted individually, and for the most part, physician bills were submitted individually by each physician provider associated with a patient's care. Bills submitted by providers have been subject to increased regulation, interpretation, and analysis by various payers, as discussed below.

Indemnity Insurers and Private Pay Patients

Indemnity insurers provide a security against loss to those who purchase policies. Indemnity insurance for health care is similar to property, casualty, or auto insurance, although specific terms may differ. Most important to this discussion is the *extent* to which payers will indemnify policyholders against loss. *Deductibles,* amounts to be satisfied before benefits are paid, and *copayments,* percentages of the total loss borne by insureds, are used to share the risk, thereby lowering insurance costs and discouraging over-utilization. Indemnity insurers continue to receive the patient's bill until they pay a specific percentage of the total bill against certain maximums; the patient is responsible for the remainder.

Private pay patients have no insurance and therefore are required to pay the total amount of charges billed.

Medicare

Medicare is a "fee-for-service" system. It pays a fee for each service provided to a covered patient.

In 1983 Medicare revamped its reimbursement system from a retrospective, cost-based model to a prospective, case-rate model based on diagnosis-related groups (DRGs). The intent of the DRG system is to create an environment in which risk is shared between the Medicare program and the hospital provider. Individual procedures and diagnoses have been identified and a weight assigned to each DRG.

The Health Care Financing Administration (HCFA) recognizes that situations differ across the country in a variety of market and environmental factors. Thus an institution-specific case index is determined, based on a number of factors (urban or rural environment and applicable wages in the area, for example). By multiplying the case rate by the case weight, the total reimbursement (subject to minor modifications) is determined. Table 6-5 (pp. 152–53) demonstrates the reimbursement methodology for Medicare as well as other payers for a sample hospital; it also lists the relative weights for all cardiovascular DRGs.

The prospective payment system recognizes that certain cases fall outside what is considered normal courses of treatment for a particular diagnosis. These patients will exceed either the maximum length of stay allowed for a DRG or the total charges identified for that DRG. The 1991 thresholds for these "outliers" has been set by HCFA as either the geometric mean of the length of stay plus the lesser of 29 days or 3 standard deviations or the greater of two times the DRG rate or $34,000.

Medicare outpatients continue to be reimbursed on a modified cost-based system, thereby requiring hospitals to continue their Medicare cost-reporting practices.

Medicaid

Medicaid is a federally mandated program that provides compensated care for the poor. Although the program is partially funded by the federal government, it is controlled by the states, with each state sharing in the funding. Medicaid funding varies widely from a cost-based system through DRG-related systems, through per diem systems to capped reimbursement amounts per hospital. It is essential, therefore, that each management team determine the reimbursement methodologies in place for Medicaid patients in its state.

Blue Cross

Blue Cross represents a significant percentage of non-Medicare and non-Medicaid patients. Because Blue Cross is managed on a local or statewide basis, the reimbursement practices of each program vary from state to state. Again, cardiovascular management personnel must be familiar with the Blue Cross payment methodologies in place within their state.

Managed Care

Managed care, a fairly new segment of the payer market, is a supplement or an alternative to conventional indemnity insurance plans. Managed care includes health maintenance organizations (HMOs), preferred provider organizations (PPOs), third-party administrators, and specialty preferred provider organizations (SPPOs). The importance of managed care varies considerably from market to market, as do the maturity and sophistication of the managed care payers within a market. By way of background, four managed care reimbursement methodologies are reviewed here: percentage discounts, per diems, case rates, and package pricing.

Percentage Discounts

The first attempt by major employers to achieve savings in the health care arena came through the negotiation of a *percentage discount,* a reduction of the total patient bill based on an agreed-on percentage. However, whereas these discounts provide a relative benefit to the payers, they ultimately do not result in true savings over time and are losing popularity. Another reason they are losing ground is that they are applied to hospital charges that are continually adjusted higher.

Table 6-5. Reimbursement by Payer Class

Charge and Reimbursement Analysis of Financial Class
Cardiovascular DRGs
Fiscal Year 1989

DRG	Financial Class	Case	Charges	Ave. Case Charge	Hospital Days	ALOS	Per Case	Estimated Reimbursement Total	Total Discount
104	Blue Cross	1	80,145	80,145	41	41.0	$26,766	$26,766	($53,379)
	Comm. Ins.	5	287,850	57,570	94	18.8	46,056	230,280	(57,570)
	PPO							0	0
	Medicaid						22,254	0	0
	Medicare	10	951,737	95,174	410	41.0	31,937	319,367	(632,370)
	Self-pay								
	Total	16	1,319,732	82,483	545	34.1	$36,026	$576,414	($743,318)
105	Blue Cross	3	99,928	33,309	27	9.0	$19,089	$57,267	($42,661)
	Comm. Ins.	6	237,441	39,574	82	13.7	31,659	189,953	(47,488)
	PPO	3	97,637	32,546	23	7.7	5,827	17,480	(80,157)
	Medicaid	4	218,805	54,701	35	8.8	18,865	75,462	(143,343)
	Medicare	21	1,621,089	77,195	456	21.7	24,417	512,760	(1,108,329)
	Self-pay								
	Total	37	2,274,900	61,484	623	16.8	$23,052	$852,922	($1,421,978)
106	Blue Cross	19	722,362	38,019	247	13.0	$22,160	$421,038	($301,324)
	Comm. Ins.	27	1,035,465	38,351	351	13.0	30,680	828,372	(207,093)
	PPO	6	234,309	39,052	78	13.0	9,880	59,280	(175,029)
	Medicaid	1	41,795	41,795	9	9.0	18,865	18,865	(22,930)
	Medicare	69	3,614,907	52,390	1,039	15.1	23,030	1,589,060	(2,025,847)
	Self-pay	3	88,621	29,540	22	7.3	23,632	70,897	(17,724)
	Total	125	5,737,459	45,900	1,746	14.0	$23,900	$2,987,512	($2,749,947)

107	Blue Cross	19	579,045	30,476	154	8.1	$16,114	$306,160	($272,885)
	Comm. Ins.	35	1,015,012	29,000	287	8.2	23,200	812,010	(203,002)
	PPO	7	303,823	43,403	62	8.9	6,731	47,120	(256,703)
	Medicaid	5	210,106	42,021	55	11.0	16,310	82,550	(127,556)
	Medicare	86	2,843,916	33,069	918	10.7	17,208	1,479,875	(1,364,041)
	Self-pay	5	118,056	23,611	34	6.8	18,889	94,445	(23,611)
	Total	157	5,069,958	32,293	1,510	9.6	$17,976	$2,822,160	($2,247,798)
112	Blue Cross	119	1,529,487	12,853	434	3.6	$6,926	$824,151	($705,336)
	Comm. Ins.	224	2,774,850	12,388	811	3.6	9,910	2,219,880	(554,970)
	PPO	19	242,853	12,782	55	2.9	2,200	41,800	(201,053)
	Medicaid	16	262,483	16,405	106	6.6	7,810	124,956	(137,527)
	Medicare	338	4,704,239	13,918	1,653	4.9	7,780	2,629,363	(2,074,676)
	Self-pay	21	341,212	16,248	109	5.2	12,999	272,970	(68,242)
	Total	737	9,855,124	13,372	3,168	4.3	$8,295	$6,113,120	($3,741,804)
	Grand Totals	1,072	24,257,173		7,592			$13,352,327	($10,904,846)

Average OHS Charge $43,081

Average OHS Reimbursement $21,609

Average Comm. Ins. Reimbursement $28,228

Per Diems

In an effort to gain more control over hospital costs, managed care providers began negotiating daily rates for various types of care. Generally referred to as *per diems,* these reimbursements reflect the average cost of care on a per day basis and differ for general medical–surgical beds and critical care beds. Depending on the rate and mix of cases referred, per diem arrangements can be beneficial to the payer, the provider, or both.

Case Rates

Given the success to date of the Medicare DRG system, there is an increasing tendency among payers to negotiate individual *case rates* for major high-cost, subspecialty procedures, such as coronary artery bypass or valve repair/replacement. This trend will continue, given its apparent capabilities to save on costs and to shift the risk of patient care management to the hospital.

Package Pricing

To streamline and simplify reimbursement, managed care companies are negotiating more *package services,* whereby all hospital and physician fees are incorporated into one "global" fee. Typically, initiated by payers, package prices not only can shift risk but also predict costs of care while eliminating individual bills from a variety of sources. (Package pricing will be discussed in greater detail later in this chapter.)

Future Patterns of Reimbursement

It is highly probable that the fee-for-service system of reimbursement, formerly popular with both payers and providers, will become less popular with payers. The rapid increase in health care costs and anxiety on the part of payers and employers will pave the way for prospective payment, risk sharing, and fixed cost pricing. This will require stronger relationships between hospitals and physicians in providing products and services to the payer communities. Specialty preferred provider organizations and some HMOs, which are developing around high-cost subspecialty services, are examples of this innovation toward prospectively established fixed cost prices that link hospitals and physician providers.

It can also be expected that, for economic and pricing reasons, efforts will continue to regionalize high-cost subspecialty services, such as cardiovascular surgery. Smaller programs will respond by accepting only routine cases that can be performed safely and economically at the local level. More difficult cases will be sent to the higher-volume regional or tertiary centers, which consequently will have high case costs based on the severity of cases. Maintaining local services built around less difficult cases is a reasonable health-planning policy because it maintains a certain standard of proficiency at that level and enables local providers to offer improved care for the more difficult or emergent cases that cannot be transported to regional centers. A predictable result would be the creation of factors to enhance the level of reimbursement to regional referral centers and/or decrease the reimbursement to those centers that perform only the more routine cases. It is possible that new DRGs will be created to account for the differences in severity levels.

The impact of resource-based relative value units (RBRVUs) and the development of ambulatory procedure DRGs (or APGs) may be significant in restructuring the type of services provided and the location of those services. The recently implemented resource-based relative value scale (RBRVS) for physician reimbursement may also have a significant impact on the types and volumes of procedures being performed.

Pricing

The cost and price for cardiovascular surgery and cardiovascular services are issues of grave concern. Because of the high incidence of cardiovascular disease and the high cost of its diagnosis and treatment, many payers have identified cardiovascular disease as the single largest component of health-related expenditures. It is also the biggest source of hospital revenue. Therefore, cardiologists and cardiac surgeons rank highest as hospital revenue sources. As more entrants participate in the cardiovascular market and new initiatives emerge for reducing the cost of cardiovascular care, attention focuses on the price of cardiovascular services, which in turn causes a new and deeper focus on the underlying costs of these services.

In many markets, the range of prices for cardiovascular surgery differs by more than 100 percent between the lowest-priced provider and the highest-priced provider. There are also substantial differences between the average price for cardiovascular surgery by region across the country. Estimates of these costs are given in table 6-6.

Within DRG 105, for example, the range of prices extends from a low of $19,718 in Vermont to a high of $80,071 in Nevada, a difference of more than 400 percent. In markets where a significant portion of the patient population comes from Medicare, Medicaid, or managed care contracts, being at the high end of this price continuum can be a problem, certainly where case price and case cost are related.

Table 6-5 arrays the distribution of cases by DRG across a payer mix matrix for a sample hospital. Note that the average case reimbursement for

Table 6-6. Discharges, Average Charges, and LOS for DRGs 104–107, 112, 124, 125: HCFA CY 1987 (age 65+)

	DRG 104			DRG 105			DRG 106		
State	Discharges	Average Charges	Average LOS	Discharges	Average Charges	Average LOS	Discharges	Average Charges	Average LOS
National	9,165	$44,437	22.4	9,890	$35,914	16.9	51,290	$31,841	17.0
Alabama	220	$49,466	20.7	225	$40,041	15.3	1,360	$31,576	14.7
Alaska	5	$99,511	37.0	5	$18,078	8.0	20	$36,661	26.3
Arizona	150	$40,666	19.3	155	$45,536	18.0	955	$34,471	16.0
Arkansas	105	$25,529	16.4	110	$22,690	15.6	925	$20,199	14.6
California	1,005	$55,622	18.2	1,370	$42,419	14.0	5,305	$43,860	15.6
Colorado	75	$44,875	19.9	90	$38,988	17.8	455	$33,552	17.0
Connecticut	185	$33,239	26.0	195	$28,635	19.7	435	$28,522	21.9
Delaware	10	$43,830	19.0	10	$55,023	28.0	40	$44,372	20.6
District of Columbia	45	$68,497	27.6	40	$62,003	25.9	340	$35,028	15.8
Florida	875	$47,310	21.4	535	$36,954	15.3	4,350	$33,888	16.3
Georgia	105	$40,137	18.2	240	$32,815	15.7	850	$27,076	15.4
Hawaii	40	$54,027	19.0	20	$28,764	14.0	160	$51,888	20.8
Idaho	5	$29,225	20.0	35	$28,592	14.9	95	$30,627	20.0
Illinois	315	$46,717	23.5	300	$39,693	16.8	2,005	$32,141	18.1
Indiana	285	$44,999	26.4	160	$33,536	14.7	1,480	$31,939	18.4
Iowa	115	$33,044	25.3	85	$25,225	14.5	830	$23,736	15.5
Kansas	110	$42,307	18.1	40	$34,943	18.0	715	$30,420	15.2
Kentucky	105	$51,489	23.2	95	$48,416	20.3	655	$29,370	18.1
Louisiana	135	$52,866	24.6	110	$36,413	15.4	850	$34,296	16.7
Maine	20	$45,326	32.5	80	$21,144	15.3	170	$24,820	21.6
Maryland	15	$30,006	19.0	205	$28,348	19.5	135	$22,525	21.1
Massachusetts	215	$55,735	28.6	335	$36,661	17.4	780	$36,412	20.2
Michigan	210	$56,169	24.5	390	$46,037	18.3	1,250	$35,679	17.6
Minnesota	310	$30,508	19.2	130	$23,960	12.5	885	$25,462	15.6
Mississippi	40	$30,446	15.1	30	$23,908	10.3	555	$22,040	14.2
Missouri	380	$37,801	20.4	270	$39,494	15.7	2,105	$29,720	16.4
Montana	20	$39,045	17.3	85	$38,648	18.2	215	$29,740	13.8
Nebraska	70	$40,020	17.1	35	$25,328	14.6	455	$29,833	15.3
Nevada	65	$82,118	22.6	55	$80,071	16.9	260	$53,042	16.6
New Hampshire	25	$51,588	34.6	25	$28,624	14.2	140	$29,178	18.1
New Jersey	190	$32,958	24.8	270	$33,543	20.1	735	$24,620	20.1
New Mexico	50	$48,683	23.9	30	$27,284	10.7	195	$25,922	11.5
New York	530	$37,439	31.7	870	$31,314	22.3	1,880	$25,201	21.6
North Carolina	190	$43,426	26.5	235	$23,479	13.9	1,445	$26,720	17.8
North Dakota	30	$41,078	24.7	45	$29,585	15.8	300	$27,917	16.8
Ohio	365	$42,965	23.2	470	$34,044	17.2	2,280	$28,744	18.2
Oklahoma	145	$37,605	19.6	75	$33,478	15.7	1,015	$27,550	16.3
Oregon	115	$36,265	18.0	130	$26,074	12.3	680	$25,666	13.1
Pennsylvania	740	$55,278	22.7	580	$42,423	15.6	3,280	$42,023	17.9
Rhode Island	15	$19,033	22.7	95	$32,778	22.8	120	$26,588	19.7
South Carolina	60	$46,050	34.6	70	$26,151	15.1	655	$23,815	16.3
South Dakota	80	$24,822	18.2	20	$25,442	18.5	260	$20,014	16.8
Tennessee	180	$43,967	23.0	155	$30,848	15.4	1,870	$29,089	18.3
Texas	570	$36,133	20.0	460	$37,241	19.9	3,885	$30,940	17.0
Utah	80	$29,610	16.1	100	$31,592	17.8	305	$20,595	13.1
Vermont	35	$46,200	30.7	25	$19,718	11.0	75	$26,342	22.8
Virginia	100	$39,485	25.3	230	$39,106	18.2	820	$30,028	16.8
Washington	190	$30,985	17.6	315	$26,153	14.4	1,010	$23,606	12.9
West Virginia	15	$53,767	22.3	45	$32,016	17.9	275	$34,798	19.4
Wisconsin	210	$40,743	25.9	205	$28,591	17.6	1,385	$23,766	18.0
Wyoming	15	$24,559	14.0	5	$20,662	10.0	45	$24,652	14.6

	DRG 107			DRG 112			DRG 124			DRG 125	
Discharges	Average Charges	Average LOS	Discharges	Average Charges	Average LOS	Discharges	Average Charges	Average LOS	Discharges	Average Charges	Average LOS
36,885	$25,806	13.2	80,970	$11,068	8.6	66,780	$ 6,511	6.3	89,990	$3,614	3.2
930	$24,735	11.4	1,690	$11,292	8.2	2,010	$6,766	6.2	2,310	$4,244	3.6
20	$20,272	10.3	15	$12,606	12.3	5	$13,414	8.0	15	$5,709	6.7
500	$31,863	14.9	1,430	$11,264	6.5	1,085	$6,135	4.9	1,375	$3,645	2.3
375	$15,294	11.0	805	$7,402	8.4	895	$4,364	5.6	1,260	$3,296	3.5
3,880	$36,017	12.5	10,090	$13,640	6.5	6,475	$8,482	5.4	4,665	$5,424	3.1
340	$26,474	12.1	800	$10,432	7.3	450	$5,614	4.6	660	$3,553	2.7
620	$19,432	14.1	915	$9,634	10.0	1,145	$7,191	8.1	1,150	$3,024	2.6
180	$27,310	15.5	105	$8,788	10.0	80	$5,341	5.3	235	$3,178	2.6
365	$26,592	11.2	540	$11,252	7.1	370	$5,807	4.2	795	$2,753	1.7
2,235	$27,724	12.7	5,950	$12,272	8.6	5,745	$6,174	5.4	6,910	$3,884	3.1
1,060	$25,654	13.0	1,750	$9,604	8.4	1,645	$6,641	5.2	1,895	$4,714	5.6
180	$41,186	14.4	200	$11,651	7.2	145	$6,200	5.0	190	$4,131	2.4
110	$18,209	10.3	190	$6,957	6.2	175	$4,602	4.1	225	$2,994	2.3
1,390	$27,923	13.9	3,215	$13,705	10.3	2,675	$8,079	7.5	4,685	$3,937	3.2
830	$29,230	14.9	2,585	$9,180	7.4	1,725	$5,989	6.9	2,900	$3,483	3.8
345	$18,670	12.0	1,365	$9,233	8.2	710	$5,467	6.8	1,045	$3,789	3.4
220	$26,940	12.3	1,115	$11,146	8.4	600	$6,301	6.8	1,090	$3,320	2.8
570	$25,881	12.3	755	$11,329	9.5	1,090	$6,025	7.1	1,300	$3,420	3.7
385	$26,572	11.9	1,565	$12,270	8.5	1,380	$6,810	5.9	1,705	$4,489	3.4
290	$18,349	14.1	230	$8,910	9.7	330	$5,943	8.8	410	$2,707	2.9
585	$16,632	12.8	1,050	$8,277	10.2	785	$5,037	6.5	1,130	$2,377	2.5
1,110	$28,479	14.9	1,700	$12,598	11.6	1,480	$7,966	8.0	1,725	$3,808	2.9
1,760	$27,769	12.7	2,540	$11,571	8.2	2,085	$7,419	6.4	2,125	$3,860	2.7
560	$21,045	11.7	1,195	$10,495	7.6	670	$5,766	5.9	1,370	$3,094	2.3
150	$21,845	13.1	615	$9,230	9.2	385	$5,407	6.5	655	$3,135	3.6
940	$24,814	12.5	3,015	$11,397	8.8	2,135	$7,048	7.1	2,830	$3,855	3.9
145	$29,730	12.0	525	$9,823	6.0	220	$5,767	4.7	460	$3,362	2.0
135	$23,348	11.9	595	$10,184	8.0	310	$7,768	6.5	405	$4,503	3.8
190	$41,501	13.3	510	$12,529	6.5	360	$7,972	5.0	210	$6,393	4.4
155	$21,878	12.1	270	$8,828	8.6	155	$4,109	4.0	285	$2,804	2.6
895	$20,000	14.9	1,820	$10,266	14.0	1,835	$5,007	7.2	2,925	$2,336	2.8
45	$35,407	16.9	360	$10,844	6.7	170	$6,919	5.5	205	$3,741	2.5
2,570	$19,835	15.2	3,830	$10,039	13.3	3,955	$6,102	7.7	4,945	$2,874	3.1
770	$19,253	12.0	1,685	$10,313	9.3	1,545	$4,930	5.8	1,875	$3,217	3.4
200	$22,710	11.2	195	$9,600	6.4	210	$6,519	6.1	575	$3,680	2.7
2,135	$24,949	14.7	4,080	$10,558	9.2	3,620	$5,788	6.0	6,210	$3,170	3.1
245	$21,119	11.3	1,175	$10,570	8.0	770	$5,969	5.9	1,345	$3,393	2.8
480	$19,180	9.7	1,140	$8,356	5.8	765	$4,698	3.8	1,095	$2,752	2.0
2,335	$29,558	12.4	4,805	$11,788	9.2	4,510	$7,875	7.2	6,205	$3,877	3.0
125	$18,919	13.4	375	$7,507	8.7	215	$5,880	8.6	340	$2,521	2.3
240	$22,703	13.3	845	$9,553	9.5	640	$5,621	7.3	530	$3,807	4.3
65	$14,421	12.5	225	$7,377	7.9	75	$7,044	7.6	240	$3,513	3.7
760	$23,945	12.7	1,630	$10,693	9.6	1,550	$6,509	7.5	3,020	$4,030	4.5
1,830	$23,565	13.6	4,860	$10,758	8.2	4,400	$6,267	5.9	5,650	$4,090	3.5
250	$17,126	10.9	545	$6,868	4.7	345	$4,640	4.0	600	$2,508	1.9
120	$21,006	19.8	140	$10,344	7.8	155	$5,774	6.2	210	$2,297	2.5
820	$29,541	15.0	1,580	$9,657	8.5	1,420	$5,818	5.8	1,810	$3,350	3.0
1,165	$20,048	11.0	1,705	$8,669	5.8	1,095	$5,805	5.2	1,000	$3,325	2.5
150	$24,717	14.2	495	$12,684	11.7	4,810	$6,297	6.7	815	$3,995	3.7
1,110	$22,635	14.9	2,085	$8,955	8.2	1,410	$5,511	6.8	3,110	$2,947	2.7
20	$18,429	8.8	70	$7,243	6.6	45	$3,838	3.4	150	$2,250	1.9

DRGs 104, 105, 106, and 107 was $21,609, which includes commercial insurance patients. The estimated reimbursement for commercial insurance was $28,228. In this example, the average case charge was $43,081. This comparison results in an average contractual allowance of approximately 50 percent. Unless this sample hospital was employing market-driven pricing practices that allowed the market (rather than the cost structure) to set the price, it can be assumed that little or no profit was generated from cardiovascular surgery and PTCA.

If hospitals like this sample case are to bring total "à la carte" case charges into the $20,000 to $25,000 range, they must develop strategies for becoming competitive in the managed care contracting environment. Payers looking to halt cost shifting increasingly will contract only with hospitals that can document a profit from the contract patients.

All effective strategies for case price reduction involve modifying physician practice patterns, which account for the principal difference in case price. Therefore, the physicians' active involvement in managing case prices will be critical. In general, historical attempts to achieve this result have failed, principally because the physicians lacked the *incentive* to change their behavior. Information and administrative admonition offer little incentive for physicians to change their ways, but linking increased patient volume to modified practice patterns can. Case 1 in chapter 11 describes a process by which this modification of physician behavior was implemented successfully.

Price-Based Competition

Hospitals compete for cardiovascular patients on the basis of the quality of service, geographic location, and price. All three factors are important, but price is of particular interest to hospital managers in their efforts to balance price with volume.

Given the current range of prices for cardiovascular surgery in certain markets nationally, there are opportunities to compete very effectively on the basis of price. Current interest in "centers of excellence" is motivated principally by payers' efforts to reduce costs rather than to improve quality— although the two can be related. Where this market condition exists, it should be aggressively exploited. Institutions in a position to do so should participate in centers of excellence programs and initiate formation of SPPOs.

Over a period of time, price differences of this magnitude will disappear as the market moves toward equilibrium. As this occurs, certain inefficient providers will be eliminated from the market. Also, certain low-cost programs with disproportionately large volumes for their service area will lose substantial volumes when the market shifts its attention in the value equation (value = price + quality + convenience) from price and clinical quality to convenience and service quality.

To position a program to compete effectively on the basis of price, managers must — as repeated throughout this book — attract high-caliber, team-oriented physicians. Although it may seem axiomatic, it is true that a competitive program cannot be structured around inferior physicians. For example, if a surgeon routinely cannot complete individual cases in less than four hours, there is nothing the rest of the team can do to reduce case costs significantly because the surgeon's patients are sicker than other surgeon's patients following surgery. On the other hand, when a surgeon's average cross-clamp time is 45 minutes or less, the program is poised to be extremely competitive.

The program must promote group unity and a desire to work toward common goals. Many notable low-cost programs are organized around a single physician (often the senior surgeon), who provides group direction, goals, and focus. Without this kind of leadership, programs can lapse into mediocrity. Program personnel do well, but the program does poorly. Those who do well are not motivated to change, and those who do not do so well cannot bring about change. Only an event outside the program, a perceived threat perhaps, can galvanize program members and bring about change.

Package Pricing

Increased competition in the cardiovascular services market, driven not only by the larger role played by managed care providers but also by their growing number, is opening the door for innovative pricing methods. As noted earlier, one such innovation is package pricing, which combines physician and hospital charges into a single price.

To arrive at a package price a hospital first must have accurate and adequate DRG cost data for their product. Previously, these data were drawn from retrospective hospital experience and then used to predict costs. It must be noted that the term *costs* in this context is used loosely in that many hospital cost-accounting systems are limited in their ability to determine accurate costs for providing various services. However, this has not stopped them from establishing per case prices — despite not knowing their profit level or even whether they cover their costs.

Because of rising concern over cost shifting, many payers will negotiate only with hospitals that demonstrate profit levels keyed to their fixed fee quotes. As always, case costs vary with physicians, and a hospital negotiating a fixed fee contract must seek alliance with the best-skilled providers if it wants to secure patient services contracts.

Selecting providers for package price contracts can be complicated by certain logistics in managing the negotiation and implementation of agreements. For example, the more physicians involved in the negotiation process, the more difficult it is for a payer to select a provider. Therefore, hospitals that can simplify the physician component – thus simplifying the selection process – have a better chance of being awarded contracts.

The hospital's objective in securing a packaged fee contract is to extract value from a relationship with a payer. This value comes from the security of volume, the profits generated from the service, and the capacity to increase volume that is associated with the contract. The greater the value expected by the providers, the more willing they will be to lower their prices, which should be decreased in relationship to specific factors:

- Size of the payer
- Capacity of the payer to modify its benefit package in order to attract patients
- Extent to which the contract represents potential new sources of business

Package price contracting involves politics and strategy. The facility that can streamline its delivery system and its organizational structure so as to allow flexibility and practice pattern efficiency will further its success in this arena.

Coding

Although *ICD-9-CM* coding expertise generally exists within the medical record department, whose responsibility it is to code all discharges, cardiovascular management must share this responsibility if reimbursement is to be maximized. Program management must become familiar with the coding process, including proper coding of diagnostic and procedure codes, supplementary (V and E) codes, linkages with other codes (*CPT-4* coding), linkages with medical and/or surgical DRGs, the relative reimbursements for each DRG (see table 6-7), the basis for assigning codes, the reimbursement associated with each code, and ultimately, the individual physician's performance in the process. Managers must also help ensure timely and accurate completion of all medical records.

A mechanism must be developed for the regular auditing of DRG-related coding along with frequent feedback to physicians and others who prepare discharge summaries. This communication plan also must include educational programs, refresher courses, bulletins, and changes in coding and writing discharge summaries. Finally, physicians must be reminded regularly of the economic importance of the process.

Financial Management for Cardiovascular Services

As discussed in chapter 5, data become information only when they are used to make decisions that lead to action that in turn brings about change. So

Table 6-7.   Cardiovascular DRGs (Diseases/Disorders of the Circulatory System)

DRG	1992 Relative Weight
Cardiovascular Surgical	
103 Heart transplant	14.0323
104 Cardiac valve procedure with pump and with cardiac cath	8.2575
105 Cardiac valve procedure with pump and without cardiac cath	6.1581
106 Coronary bypass with cardiac cath	5.4470
107 Coronary bypass without cardiac cath	4.9616
108 Cardiothoracic procedures, except valve and coronary bypass, with pump	5.9600
109 Cardiothoracic procedures without pump (no longer valid)	0.0000
115 Permanent cardiac pacemaker implant with AMI or CHF	3.6795
116 Permanent cardiac pacemaker implant without AMI or CHF	2.4973
117 Cardiac pacemaker replacement and revision except pulse generator replacement only	1.2743
Cardiac Medical	
118 Cardiac pacemaker pulse generator replacement only	1.6957
121 Circulatory disorders with AMI or CV complications, discharged alive	1.6210
122 Circulatory disorders with AMI without CV complications, discharged alive	1.1667
123 Circulatory disorders with AMI, expired	1.3920
124 Circulatory disorders except AMI with cardiac cath and complex diagnosis	1.1973
125 Circulatory disorders except AMI with cardiac cath without complex diagnosis	0.7387
126 Acute and subacute endocarditis	2.8874
127 Heart failure and shock	1.0070
129 Cardiac arrest	1.2551
132 Atherosclerosis with C.C.	0.7312
133 Atherosclerosis without C.C.	0.5342
134 Hypertension	0.5663
135 Cardiac congenital and valvular disorders, age = 70 and/or Dx 2	0.8770
136 Cardiac congenital and valvular disorders, age 18–69 without Dx 2	0.5434
137 Cardiac congenital and valvular disorders, age 0–17	0.6239
138 Cardiac arrhythmia and conduction disorders, age = 70 and/or Dx 2	0.8211
139 Cardiac arrhythmia and conduction disorders, age F without Dx 2	0.5149
140 Angina pectoris	0.6226
141 Syncope and collapse, age = 70 and/or Dx 2	0.6950
142 Syncope and collapse, age F without Dx 2	0.5006
143 Chest pain	0.5118
Vascular Surgical	
110 Major reconstructive vascular procedures, age = 70 and/or Dx 2	4.2703
111 Major reconstructive vascular procedures, age F without Dx 2	2.3980
112 Vascular procedures except major reconstruction	2.0163
113 Amputation for circulatory system disorders except upper limb and toe	2.6925
114 Upper limb and toe amputation for circulatory system disorders	1.5499
119 Vein ligation and stripping	0.9379
120 Other O.R. procedures on the circulatory system	2.0736
Vascular Medical	
128 Deep vein thrombophlebitis	0.7906
130 Peripheral vascular disorders, age = 70 and/or Dx 2	0.9118
131 Peripheral vascular disorders, age F without Dx 2	0.5882
144 Other circulatory diagnoses with Dx 2	1.0888
145 Other circulatory diagnosis without Dx 2	0.6454

it is with financial management, which implies change through analysis of data and information that guide the cardiovascular services manager toward sound financial decisions — one of which has to do with developing a budget. The manager calls on a variety of sources and experts for the information, which, once accumulated, is disseminated to key physicians, other managers, and administrators who will be involved in the budget development process.

Budget Development

One function of financial management is to prepare an annual budget, a financial road map for the future. The cardiovascular manager participates in this process by predicting monthly units of service, revenue by unit of service, expense by expense category, and account by cost center. Some systems provide for a flexible or volume-based budget that changes as the activity or the program, department, or service changes. Such a budget provides for the differences in expense levels that can be accounted for as a result of the difference between fixed, semivariable, and variable expenses. It is also obvious that revenue generated is related directly to the volume of activity within a particular service.

The budgeting process is also a means of requesting the allocation of resources for special services such as capital equipment, acquisition, marketing campaign development, facility expansion and renovation, and so on.

Capital Expenditure Analysis

Cardiovascular services require a commitment to capital expenditures and equipment. From time to time equipment must be repaired, replaced, added to, or substituted with more recent technology. A request for allocation of budget dollars to acquire capital equipment or expand or renovate space must be understood within the context of limited resources versus return on investment. Due to dwindling resources, hospitals are under tremendous budgetary pressure and thus have fewer dollars to invest. Consequently, programs and services must compete vigorously for these scarce resources.

To secure approval for capital expenditures, planners must understand the political process behind funds allocation. Those responsible for awarding capital budgets are concerned with staying under a certain capital threshold and investing in capital expenditures that will produce the greatest return to the institution. Usually this is done by weighing *opportunity costs,* those costs represented by all the lost opportunities from alternative investments that *could have been made.*

The manager must make a case that the capital investment is a benefit to the program and a wise financial investment. Demonstrating the latter means being able to document the differential cash flow associated with the investment. *Differential cash flow* is an analysis of how cash will flow to the institution as a result of spending the money to acquire the capital improvement. Therefore, the capital request must document the amount of the investment, the amount of improved revenues, and/or reduced costs that constitute the improved cash flow over the life of the investment, and then calculate the return that these improved cash flows represent in relationship to the investment. These cash flows must also take into account the time value of money through a computation that determines the present value of the investment dollars. In so doing, the discounted rate of return or the internal rate of return will result from this analysis of discounted cash flows. Such a process should also take into account, through a subjective discussion, the risk associated with the investment.

Cost, Volume, and Quality Management

It has been contended that large-volume programs produce a higher quality of service when measured in terms of morbidity and mortality and that large volume has a positive effect on case cost. However, this is not always true.

Regardless of the program's volume, management must be concerned with managing costs and maintaining program quality, whether measured by morbidity, mortality, or other quantitative factors. Small-volume programs in particular must control case cost and outcome to ensure program viability and success.

Quality outcome affects the financial viability of the program, both in terms of its market viability and its ability to minimize outliers; proper patient selection minimizes outliers by enhancing mortality and morbidity outcome (patient selection alone may not satisfactorily manage case cost). Therefore, programs such as standard treatment protocol (STP) must be implemented so that case costs can be managed effectively with and through physician participants. With STPs and proper case selection and management, even small-volume programs can be profitable.

Decision Support Data

Data systems, historically called financial information systems or management information systems, are increasingly being referred to as *decision support systems*. Flexible systems help decision makers analyze data.

A wealth of data is available in the typical hospital setting. Thus the decision maker must determine what information is *necessary* rather than what information is *available*. Elements of successful decision support systems include the following:

- Volume by procedure
- Volume by procedure by financial class
- Volume by physician

- Average charges by physician
- Average reimbursement by physician
- Average length of stay by physician
- Average case time by physician
- Major supply costs

Much of these data can be developed into a cost/charge model wherein a typical case is modeled on the basis of average charges, from which average costs are determined. Such a system can be applied on a physician-by-physician basis to assist individual physicians in modifying their practice patterns relative to resource consumption.

Case Cost Management

In the current mature cardiovascular market, competition centers more than ever on the hospital's cost. Management of case costs has become a critical factor that every program must address. Historically, cost management revolved around controlling personnel utilization, overtime, and supplies. Now, it is imperative that the goal of comprehensive resource consumption management be to analyze and transform clinical practices so that patient services are provided efficiently *and* cost-effectively. This means developing STPs — those conventions of care based on careful analysis of the best clinical practices, balanced with careful attention to resource consumption.

By creating a multidisciplinary approach to developing STPs, the hospital can document the accepted method of patient care, ensure delivery of high-quality care, and begin to manage case costs by specifying what tests, procedures, drugs, and so forth, are part of the standard and thus believed to be cost-effective. Only by analyzing current resource consumption proactively, determining costs, and establishing the best care standards can hospitals manage their costs successfully.

Summary

Sound financial management is critical to the success of any cardiovascular program. It is important for the CVS manager to be well-versed in basic financial concepts. In assessing a new or expanded program's financial feasibility, a computerized model is recommended for generating projections that help predict outcome based on specific assumptions. Another measure of financial feasibility is whether a proposed program or service can generate spin-off revenue for the hospital. In addition to being financially feasible, a planned program also must be operationally, politically, and strategically feasible. The feasibility model also can be applied to financial performance of an existing program whose profitability is measured by the income (P & L) statement, that is, *do revenues exceed expenses?*

To attain maximum profit, cost control must be a priority—cost of inventory and supplies, personnel, operations, and so forth. In adopting product/service line management, managers can monitor case cost and apply other innovative approaches to cost reduction (cross-training, substitution, supply standardization, per unit cost analysis, and the like).

Financial managers for cardiovascular programs must know basic accounting so that they can interpret financial reporting statements, thereby detecting problems and implementing necessary changes.

Reimbursement methods are changing in response to increased payer regulation, interpretation, and demand, all of which fuels competition among providers. The results are reimbursement innovations such as health care indemnity policies; Medicare's DRG-based system (a move away from its retrospective cost-based system); and Medicaid's multiple payment systems (DRG based, cost based, per diem, reimbursement caps). Managed care plans—HMOs, PPOs, TPAs, SPPOs—provide at least four payment options: percentage discounts, per diems, cost rates, and package pricing.

Fee-for-service reimbursement will continue to lose ground with payers due to soaring health care costs. This trend will mandate closer relationships between physicians and hospitals. Furthermore, because of the prevalence of cardiovascular disease, cardiovascular programs are one of the biggest sources of hospital revenues—another reason hospitals must curtail competition between themselves and physicians. Finally, as competition increases among providers, which are already hard-pressed to find ways to cut costs, providers will need to seek out the top physicians so as to compete for patient services contracts with payers.

Within individual hospital settings, CV services program managers will be forced to compete with other programs for shrinking budget dollars. Therefore, CV managers must understand not only budget politics and strategies, but also how to control cost, volume, and quality; defend financial management decisions with accurate support data; and manage case cost.

Chapter 7

Cardiovascular Surgery Program Planning

Deciding whether to add invasive cardiology services or cardiovascular surgery depends on a variety of factors. Developing a cardiac catheterization laboratory can appear straightforward compared with adding a complex program such as cardiovascular surgery. This chapter focuses on the more complex process of implementing cardiovascular surgery and invasive cardiology services, although the methods described here can be applied to a cardiac catheterization laboratory as well.

Few services affect the total organization as much as cardiovascular surgery does. Consequently, the development and implementation processes must involve representatives from the entire organization, although some departments may be affected more than others. The grass-roots process outlined here involves representatives from key departments and a series of subcommittees and task forces whose responsibility will be to ensure efficient use of staff time during this stage.

As underscored numerous times throughout this book, physicians are central players in the development of clinical programs. Skilled and motivated cardiac surgeons, cardiac anesthesiologists, and invasive cardiologists should serve in leadership roles throughout the implementation process as well.

Recruiting the Surgeon

The impetus to implement cardiovascular surgery typically comes from cardiologists and hospital administrators as the result of invasive cardiologists who move into markets that previously lacked regular access to cardiac catheterization. Because procedures are becoming increasingly interventional, it is harder to recruit new cardiologists to the market without the lure of a laboratory in which interventional procedures can be performed. Furthermore, interventional cardiology is lucrative for cardiologists as well as for hospitals. Referral sources also pressure the diagnostic-only catheterization laboratory because many referring physicians send their patients to a full-service center.

Too often, initial planning fails to push for early selection of the cardiovascular surgeon and the surgical team, although both are key players. In that cardiovascular surgery services will compete on the basis of quality, cost, and accessibility—with accessibility favoring smaller developing programs—new programs must offer services that not only are priced competitively, but also can hold their own with competitors in terms of quality. Both conditions will hinge on the surgeon, not the market, the cardiologists, or the hospital.

In highly competitive urban and suburban settings, selection of the cardiac surgeon may be even more critical, because a surgeon in proximity to a large referral center may "lose points" on convenience. Thus, a very competent or "star" surgeon may be needed to alter referral patterns. Whether this is possible depends principally on the number of "loyal" cardiologists who support program development and the degree to which the market or community supports the physicians.

If the planning process must begin without a cardiac surgeon, an agreement should be reached to proceed only up to a certain point because many of the facility and equipment issues need to be "signed off" by a surgeon in order to avoid costly mistakes or duplication.

Also, if it is necessary to proceed without a surgeon on hand initially, an alternative is to affiliate with an existing cardiovascular surgery group. This arrangement offers some advantages—for both new programs and established referral groups—over recruiting a single surgeon. For example:

- In a start-up situation, long on-call and vacation coverage hours could discourage a surgeon-recruit, whereas affiliation with a group would ensure round-the-clock coverage.
- Affiliation can minimize risk because the group brings an already-established quality and cost record, so that data on practice patterns and resource consumption are immediately available for documentation and verification.
- Many start-ups join groups that themselves are experiencing (or facing) volume declines due to increased competition. Affiliation can pump new blood into the anemic group (so to speak) as well as help the new program by:
    - Avoiding costs associated with recruitment (for example, identifying and relocating a surgeon)
    - Minimizing the need to provide salary guarantees

- Affiliation brings new program management into contact with a large pool of physicians more readily.
- Any one group surgeon experiencing low volume could rotate through the higher-volume program from time to time to sharpen his or her skills, perform the needed number of cases during start-up, increase personal volume, and learn new techniques as they become available.
- In terms of public relations, affiliation with an established group can ward off or counter negative publicity about a "low-volume program."
- Staff for the new program will be trained directly by the new (group) surgeon in his or her specific techniques.

(Affiliating with existing programs is discussed later in this chapter.)

The selection of a surgeon or a group is a critical element in the program's success. In contracting for services, care should be taken to address the following issues:

- How would the surgeon's contract be canceled? By whom?
- Would cancellation create problems with (or for) the medical staff?
- What would it cost to cancel?
- Must the surgeon agree to leave the community or be free to continue practicing?
- What interim arrangements could be made to keep the program operating through another recruitment process?

A cardiac surgeon rarely is recruited without being offered some incentive; for example, a typical recruitment package may include a salary guarantee of up to $500,000 (sometimes more), moving expenses, and start-up costs. Some hospitals offer a medical director's fee, although this is more common in the early stages of the program when administrative demands on the surgeon are at a peak. Any such incentives should be carefully reviewed by a knowledgeable health care attorney.

In some settings, recruitment costs and guarantees may be incurred with the cardiac anesthesiologist or the perfusionist. This will depend in large measure on the structure and capability of the existing anesthesia department.

Preparing the Business Plan

Once it has been concluded that adding cardiovascular surgery is financially, operationally, politically, and strategically feasible, a strategic planning process can be initiated. This is done by completing a written business plan. Appendix A is a sample business plan for the implementation of cardiovascular surgery and invasive cardiology services. Appendix B is a sample strategic business plan useful for any cardiovascular service or program.

Business plan preparation should include representatives of major departments that will be affected by cardiovascular surgery: administration, nursing, critical care, surgery, cardiology, central services, emergency room, pharmacy, respiratory care, and facilities management. Representatives from other departments will be appropriate as dictated by local needs and conditions, keeping in mind that the size of the planning committee must be kept under control. A steering committee, called the *cardiovascular services planning committee* (CSPC), is recommended and will have primary strategic oversight responsibility for the process. Also known as the oversight committee, the CSPC typically is chaired by a member of senior management and is composed of no more than seven members. The committee also must include one representative each from cardiology and cardiac surgery (*if* the surgical team has been identified). The CSPC will be discussed in more detail later in this chapter.

The business planning process must culminate in consensus among the key players regarding *what must be done, in what order, and according to what schedule.* These agreements, together with other detailed documents, form the business plan itself.

The plan is a fluid document, subject to change as new information becomes available and as implementation progresses. It also can be used as a reference point for tracking the implementation process.

Generally speaking, the business plan should include at least six sections (described in the following sections):

1. Executive summary
2. Program description and market analysis
3. Start-up requirements
4. Marketing strategies
5. Program management and organization
6. Operations

The business plan also must specify a proposed time line that takes into consideration construction, staff recruitment, and implementation.

Executive Summary

The executive summary highlights the results of the planning process by identifying in simple terms the scope of the project, its objectives, resources required, key strategic variables that ensure project success, and the time frame for project completion. The executive summary serves to introduce newcomers to the project, and it forces those writing the plan to identify the key elements that will lead to the program's success.

Program Description and Market Analysis

The program description and market analysis sections differentiate components of the program. Whereas cardiac surgery programs share many similarities, each program will be different in how it relates to supplementary services, outreach programs, affiliation with existing providers, and the community. The cardiac surgeon, for example, may be moving from a local program or may be part of an existing nearby program. This situation will be entirely different from a hospital that embarks on the planning process with strong medical community support and the active involvement of the invasive cardiologists but with no cardiac surgeon identified yet.

The cardiovascular program will be successful only if it is based on need and opportunity that are identified accurately within the market; that is, it is market based. The program description section of the business plan therefore must address the structure, elements, and characteristics of the market.

The intent of the cardiovascular program will be to penetrate the primary and secondary markets for cardiac surgery to the extent possible. The better the planning participants analyze the market—demographics, current referral patterns, demand projections, service gaps, and the like—the more likely it is that the program will be successful.

Start-Up Requirements

The business plan must also address program start-up requirements. Because the business plan is frequently used to request funding from the hospital board or other funding agencies, this section will address issues pertaining to start-up operations: human resources, plant/location, facilities, hours, physician referrals, organization, and timetable.

In the start-up phase of a cardiovascular surgery program, plant and equipment needs must be defined clearly. For example, a review of the project's financial requirements should include a description of capital requirements: new construction, renovation, support system (electrical, heating, ventilating, air-conditioning, and so on), upgrades required, new equipment, financing sources, inventory buildup costs, and operating capital needs.

Starting a program of this nature will also have implications for medical staff, who therefore should be involved in this phase. The hospital's purpose and intent with respect to the program should be discussed with the staff; any objections should be addressed in the context of their potential impact on the hospital. For example, members of the surgical staff often are concerned with the effect such a program will have on surgery facilities, scheduling, or staffing. Failure to deal effectively with these issues could be costly in terms of support and cooperation from this constituency.

Many states require a hospital to modify its license prior to initiating cardiovascular surgery. Other states enforce regulation and compliance through certificate-of-need (CON) requirements. Licensure and regulation should be addressed at some length in the business plan, as should other legal issues that may be unique to the hospital or the environment.

Marketing Strategy

Marketing strategy outlined in the business plan must go beyond describing promotional activities (although certainly these are important ingredients). In a competitive market driven principally by physician referral (and increasingly by payer contracts), the marketing strategy must focus on these issues. Therefore, the business plan should include the following:

- A review of all key physician referral sources, with an estimation of their individual volume of cardiovascular patients and some analysis of their current referral practice
- A physician-by-physician plan for maintaining or altering current referral practices
- A review of all payers (PPOs or SPPOs, for example), including major employers, and a description of their present referral practices if any, as well as anticipated changes or payment modification
- A plan to reach each major payer group through contracting and education
- A detailed plan to manage relations with referral sources that are better than those of the competition

Cardiovascular surgery programs benefit from effective promotional campaigns and a positive public image, which leads to direct patient referrals. The more difficult issues related to positioning the program, however, lie within the medical and payer communities. Additional information regarding appropriate marketing strategy formation from this viewpoint is found in chapter 8.

Management and Organization

Program management and organization must be detailed in depth. This section of the business plan will address not only management of the implementation process, but also changes to be made in the organizational and management structures — for example, specific reporting relationships or any changes in the organizational flowchart. At the same time it must be recognized that as new positions are created, organizational structure must be revamped.

A facility that is adding cardiac surgery may not have selected an administrator, in which case recruitment is in order. Meanwhile, plans must be laid out for interim management pending selection of a credentialed cardiovascular administrator. In smaller hospitals, the addition of cardiac surgery has a stronger ripple effect; that is, the cardiovascular services administrator can affect not only the management structure but also the administrative structure.

Operations

Details of the operations of the new surgery or expanded special care units will be outlined rather than completely defined. This is because the purpose of the implementation process is to structure the framework and then address specific issues (policies and procedures, equipment and space, reassessment of various service capacities, and so on).

Adding cardiovascular surgery often results in a patient volume that exceeds the capacity of some hospital systems. For example, if direct care (such as telemetered beds for postoperative patient care) or indirect care (such as the radiology department's performing portable chest films) will be required, a facility must know that it can provide these support services should the program be added. Each department must assess the impact of the projected caseload and report any concerns to the planning committee.

Project Phasing

Some projects may be implemented in phases, for example, by adding a catheterization laboratory as the first phase and cardiovascular surgery as the second phase. The phasing section of the business plan should specify the components of each phase, a timeline for implementation, and any target volumes that might need to be reached in an early phase before going on to the next phase.

Financial Projections

Detailed financial projections should be incorporated into the business plan. A basic model is provided in table 6-1 of the preceding chapter.

Program Evaluation

A monitoring methodology that tracks program performance should be included in the business plan. Targets should be established for volumes, costs, quality/outcomes, income, and so on, and a mechanism (management reporting system) for tracking actual performance versus targeted performance should be instituted.

Implementing Cardiovascular Surgery and Invasive Cardiology Services

As mentioned earlier, an oversight committee, made up of key administrative, management, and medical staff members, is called the cardiovascular services planning committee (CSPC). As shown in figure 7-1, the CSPC (generally chaired by the program coordinator) has overall responsibility for project implementation. The coordinator should be able to devote at least 50 percent of his or her time to the project and be empowered with decision-making authority.

Figure 7-1.   Schematic of CVS Development Program

Cardiovascular Services Planning Committee (CSPC)

• Has primary programmatic strategic responsibility
• Considers cardiovascular services
• Oversees the activities of the cardiovascular services work group
• Meets semimonthly or as needed
• Is composed of key administrative, management, and medical staff members and project manager

Cardiovascular Surgery Work Group (CSWG)

• Chaired by project manager
• Chair sits on CV services planning committee
• Membership includes task force chairs
• Responsible to planning committee
• Primary function will be to serve as a monitor and clearinghouse for the work of the task forces
• Will develop a master schedule based on the plans and timetables submitted by each task force
• Will meet as necessary

Implementation Task Forces

• Chair sits on CSWG
• Interdepartmental membership
• CSWG chair is ex officio member
• Appropriate medical director(s) members available
• Other physicians added as needed
• Submit work plan and timetable to CSWG
• Submit written reports/minutes to CSWG to document progress
• Meet as needed

The CSPC focuses on major strategic and fundamental issues to be addressed throughout the project and may function as an operating committee after implementation. Not only will the CSPC advise top hospital management on all aspects of developmental decisions to be made over the course of the project, it will be responsible for a network of related task forces and subcommittees that are ultimately responsible for departmental activities. This committee also will network with colleagues at other facilities to gain access to information needed to complete implementation.

Reporting to the oversight committee is the operations implementation group, referred to here as the *cardiovascular surgery work group* (CSWG). The CSWG, which focuses on the numerous details faced at the departmental level to prepare and implement these new services, should include the project coordinator and three or four key management staff members to function as task force chairpersons.

Each department will establish an implementation plan under the guidance of the cardiovascular surgery work group. These departments will be organized into at least four implementation task forces to be chaired by members of the CSWG. Most departments will establish a subcommittee, chaired by their task force representative, to accomplish the tasks outlined per the committee's schedule (see figure 7-2).

Although all cardiovascular programs share some similarities, each program is unique in certain aspects: its preference of physicians, surgeons, and other staff members; program space allocation and adjacency to other key services; location; the practice patterns and standards of care applied by area physicians; the equipment available for use in the program; and the unique market area in which the program is based. Program design will synthesize the expectations of a multidisciplinary (and diverse) team into a single, unified cardiovascular program. Value decisions about facility renovation, the location of various facilities, the use of physicians, and so on, emerge only as the planning team takes shape.

A "grass-roots" implementation process ensures that the entire organization will have input into the plan design so as to generate the level of interest, enthusiasm, and support needed for the successful implementation of such a complex project as cardiac surgery. At the same time, control must be maintained to ensure that efforts are properly channeled and that no gaps exist in the plan.

Physicians — principally the cardiologists, the cardiovascular surgeons, and the cardiac anesthesiologists — should be intimately involved in the operational planning process because they have such a tremendous impact on how the program ultimately functions. Their "stamp of approval" validates the final product and facilitates implementation. Their involvement at this stage also enhances the likelihood that they will *remain involved* throughout the program.

Overseeing the grass-roots process primarily involves monitoring the activities and results of the various work groups and task forces to ensure that they continue to meet objectives. This responsibility rests with the CSPC and the program coordinator.

Staffing Requirements

As implementation progresses, new skills will be required of the clinical and technical staff. Human resources management will need to determine pay scales and job descriptions for new positions as well as revise or upgrade current ones. This should be done in consultation with the departmental subcommittees.

Changes will be required in the management structure, principally in the area of overseeing operations and marketing this new service. Expanding the surgery staff, adding a new and dedicated CSICU, adding monitored beds, and enhancing the cardiology department all could affect organizational structure. Often, one manager is assigned (or recruited) to oversee expansion.

Figure 7-2.   CVS Development Program Implementation Task Force Schedule

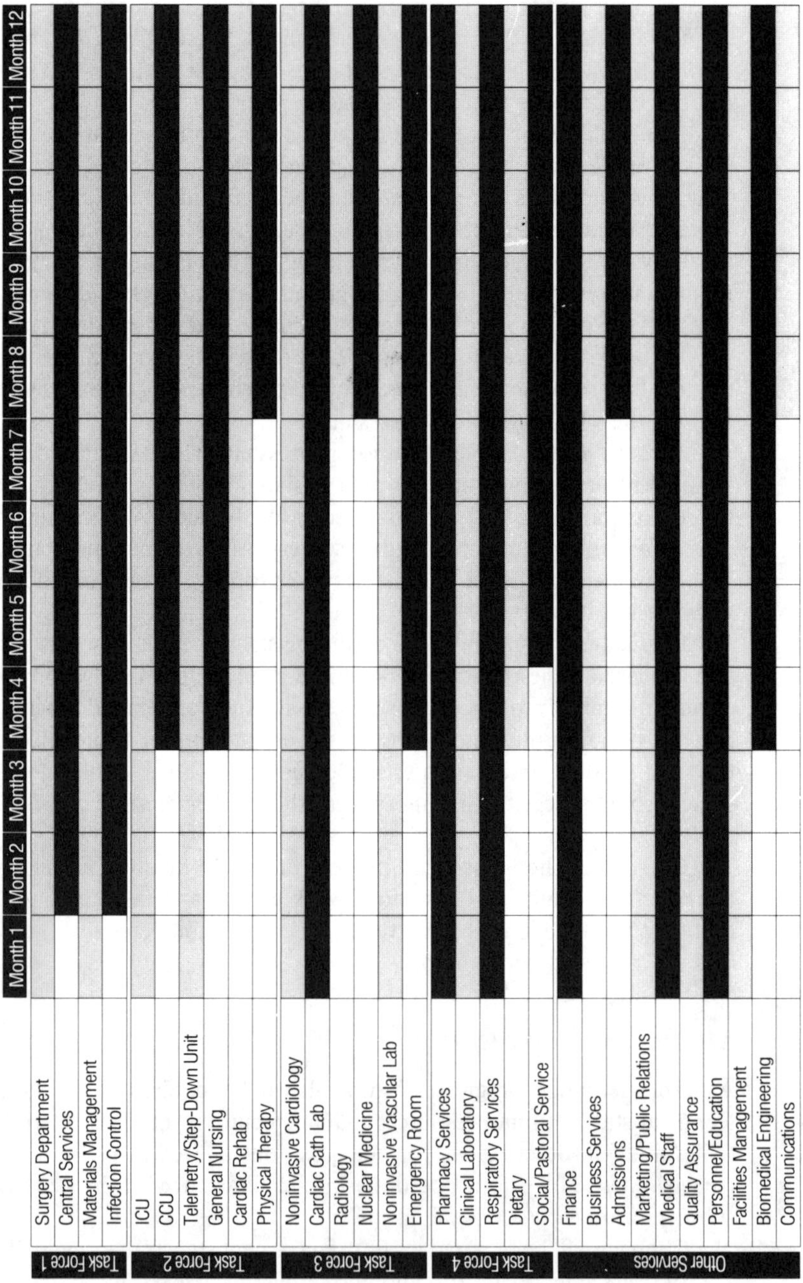

Facilities and Equipment

Significant facility renovation and upgrading, as well as a substantial addition of capital equipment, may be required; this process may require three years or more to complete. The facilities plan, including capital equipment, must be closely monitored by the CSWG, with every effort made to ensure that the project is completed on schedule, because time, strategically speaking, is of the essence. An outside construction manager should be appointed to work closely with the project coordinator, the architect, and contractor.

As will be discussed in chapter 10, procurement of equipment will depend on a strong working relationship between the project coordinator and the materials manager. This will ensure that all equipment specifications are met, that reasonable prices are secured, and that timely orders are placed.

Licensure and Compliance

In states requiring hospital license modification, the application process should commence approximately six months before expected project completion. This will be accomplished by contacting the state health care licensing agency and requesting a review of the development process to date. Forms may need to be filled out, and a visual inspection is usually part of the licensure process. Some states regulate facility size, adjacency, staffing, medical direction, equipment, and other factors.

Each departmental task force will be responsible for ensuring that applicable sections of the state regulations are reviewed and implemented as well as making necessary revisions to policies, procedures, and overall operations to ensure compliance with all pertinent JCAHO requirements — assuming the hospital is seeking accreditation.

Departmental Implementation Task Forces

Most hospital departments will have some responsibility for preparing for the addition of cardiovascular surgery. For some departments this preparation will be simple and easily accomplished; others will face a more challenging task. The creation of department implementation task forces that report to the CSWG provides a method of distributing the development and implementation work load and input throughout the hospital while providing the oversight necessary to ensure timely and well-prepared program start-up.

It is recommended that the departments affected be organized into four task forces, each with a chair who coordinates the activities of his or her group. Each chair should be a member of the CSWG. Usually, the following departments are organized into four task forces:

- Surgery
- Central services
- Materials management
- Infection control
- Nursing
- ICU
- CCU
- Telemetry
- Cardiac rehabilitation
- Physical therapy
- Cardiology
- Radiology
- Nuclear medicine
- Emergency services
- Pharmacy
- Laboratory
- Respiratory care
- Dietary services
- Social services
- Postal services

Other departments that may be included are:

- Finance
- Business services
- Admissions
- Marketing
- Public relations
- Medical staff office
- Quality assurance
- Personnel
- Education
- Facilities
- Biomedical engineering
- Communication

Departments not included in a task force will be responsible to the project coordinator and will be expected to prepare an implementation program notebook (described in the next section). This notebook serves as the control vehicle for the project coordinator.

Each task force will begin its activities by completing the task force organization worksheet (figure 7-3). This worksheet is intended to serve as a statement of purpose that clarifies task force organization and duties and acts as a control mechanism for the CSWG.

Whereas each task force or subcommittee has unique duties and responsibilities, some are common to most task forces. The worksheet shown in figure 7-3 is supplemented by the checklist shown in figure 7-4. These two documents will provide a starting point for necessary task force or subcommittee activities, such as the following:

- Identify necessary actions to prepare each department/service for new cardiovascular services.

Figure 7-3. CVS Development Program Task Force Organization Worksheet

Task Force: _____

  Chair: _____

  Membership: _____

_____

_____

_____

Frequency of Meetings: _____

Design/Planning Issues: _____

(Phase 1) _____

_____

Development Issues: _____

(Phase 2) _____

_____

Implementation Issues: _____

(Phase 3) _____

_____

Maintenance Issues: _____

(Phase 4; ongoing) _____

_____

- Provide a uniform method for project development with each department/service.
- Provide a uniform method for reporting of each department/service's progress.
- Develop a detailed implementation plan that guides each service through the process.

Figure 7-4. Task Force and Subcommittee Responsibility Checklist

Task Force _____

Department _____

Form Completed By _____

Date _____

1. Review impact issues and make appropriate revisions; attach revised copy.

2. Describe the implications of this service from the perspective of the following:
   a. State health code requirements
   b. JCAHO accreditation
   c. Other licensure or certification

3. Identify an appropriate contact person at resource hospital(s) for this function.

4. Outline in detail impact this program will have on staffing:
   a. Prepare revised staffing plan
   b. Prepare justifications for additional personnel
   c. Prepare appropriate job descriptions
   d. Explain any unique recruitment difficulties that are anticipated
   e. Identify any substantial training implications

5. Describe the impact this program will have on current facilities and equipment:
   a. Prepare description of additional equipment
   b. Prepare justification as appropriate

6. Identify new or revised hospital policies and procedures that will be required. Secure copies of resource hospital(s) documents as appropriate.

7. Identify new or revised departmental policies and procedures that will be required. Secure resource hospital(s) documents as appropriate.

8. Identify anticipated interdepartmental procedures to be modified or issues that will have to be resolved.

9. Outline modifications to be made in the department's quality assurance program.

10. Submit appropriate revisions to the Safety and Disaster Manual.

11. Develop modifications to inventory or regular supplies to be used in the program.

12. Identify any impact on the medical staff.

13. Outline preventive maintenance requirements.

14. Recommend changes to the charge master.

15. List any changes or additions necessary in the chart of accounts (cost centers, subaccounts, and so forth).

- Distribute development tasks throughout the organization so that all managers and supervisors are involved at an early stage.
- Assist in disseminating information regarding the new program throughout the organization to gain support of all employees and medical staff.
- Allow task force or subcommittee to "micromanage" each department's or service's stage of development.
- Provide the basis for each department's or service's individualized issues/plan/timetable document.

Each task force is then responsible for preparing and maintaining a timetable that includes all major activities and for reporting progress to the work group regularly.

Like the business plan, the implementation process must be fluid and dynamic so that it can respond to the changing environment. The process described here reflects the degree of difficulty and complexity involved. It also provides sufficient flexibility to make allowances for organizational strengths and weaknesses.

Implementation Schedule

A project implementation schedule will consist of four integrated schedules:

1. Master schedule
2. Facilities schedule
3. Equipment schedule
4. Implementation task force schedule

The implementation task force schedule (figure 7-2) dictates the schedule for all task forces. Each task force and departmental subcommittee will establish its own schedule and govern its own work pace. The initiation of each group's planning activities should be phased so that groups with fewer tasks will not complete their work "too soon." If this happens, the process must be repeated because employees forget, transfer, or leave the hospital. These timetables should then be integrated into the master schedule, which will be updated regularly.

Separate schedules should also be prepared for facility renovations and equipment acquisition. Both of these activities can involve significant lead time and must be addressed early on in the process. These schedules should also be incorporated into the master schedule.

Implementation Materials

A variety of supplementary implementation resources will need to be developed throughout the project (in addition to the forms found in figures 7-3 and 7-4). These include staffing plans, job descriptions, hospital budget forms, staff addition requests, equipment lists, new departmental policies and procedures, staff education plans, revised supply requirements, and purchase requisitions.

A description of the process and the relationships of the various committees should also be included in the implementation materials. These relationships are subject to revision as additional information becomes available regarding work flow.

Involvement of Other Departments in Implementation

Each hospital department — including those not on task forces — should develop an implementation program. These programs will list how each department or service would be affected by the cardiovascular surgery program and what steps the department would take to prepare for implementation. These steps will detail activities such as outlining when personnel will be hired, revising inventory requirements, securing approval for new positions, and so forth. Each department or subcommittee should create an implementation program notebook, which will contain the following sections:

- Complete list of all anticipated program effects
- Detailed plan to address issues such as facilities, equipment, space, staff, training, supplies, storage, interdepartmental interactions and relationships, policies and procedures, clinical protocols, medical directorship, medical staff, staffing plans, training resources, and so forth
- Detailed implementation/preparation schedule addressing all issues identified above
- Departmental policies, procedures, and protocols collected from other hospitals
- Meeting agendas and minutes (biweekly meetings for high-impact areas)
- Progress reports for distribution to task force chair (to be reviewed regularly by CSWG)
- Materials, information, and literature regarding equipment and supplies required by the new program
- Other accurate and timely information so the department remains up-to-date

After compiling a comprehensive list of preparatory steps based on the checklist in figure 7-4, each department should prepare a detailed schedule for the steps required to complete implementation (figure 7-5). The use of a questionnaire similar to the one found in appendix C may provide additional insight into this process. These steps and the schedule for each department will then be reviewed by the department's task force chair and reported

Figure 7-5.   CVS Development Program Implementation Schedule/Timetable

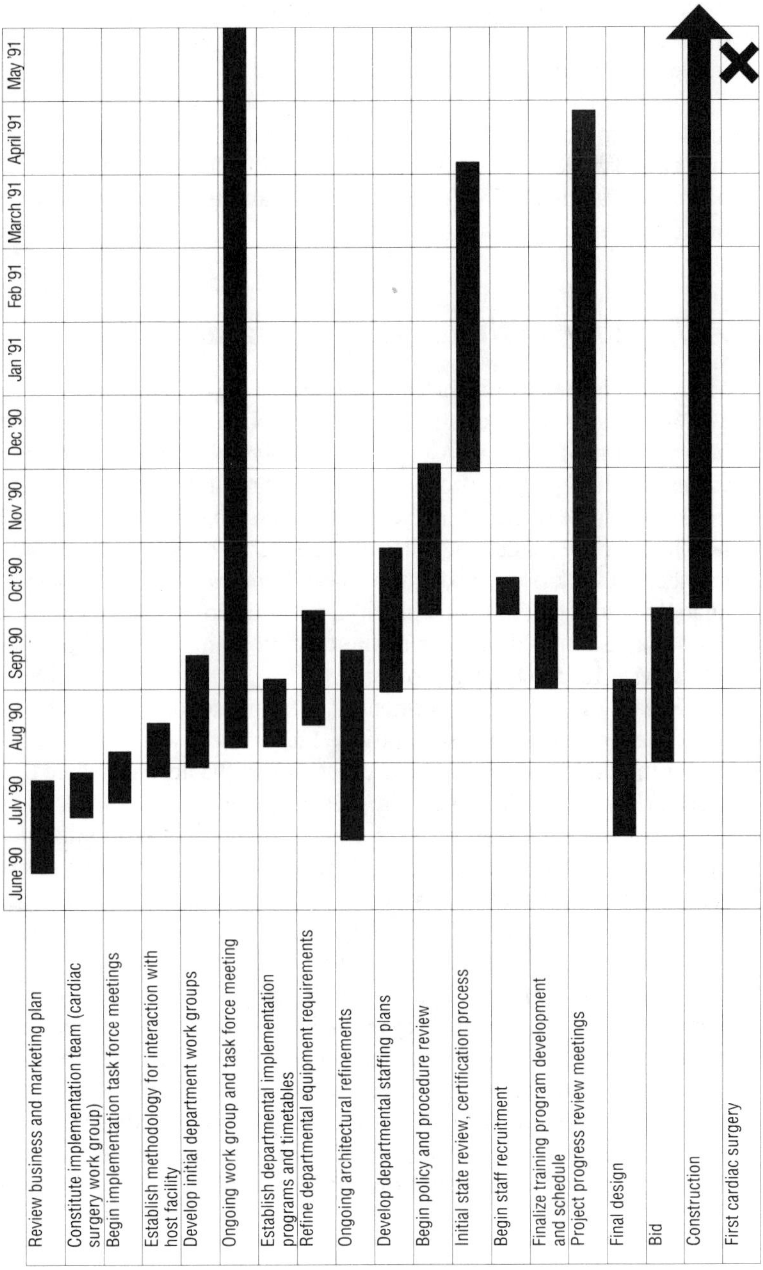

to the CSWG during regular meetings. These progress reports then continue throughout the implementation period (until cardiovascular surgery is fully implemented and all phases are complete).

Task force chairs should meet regularly with each departmental implementation team (made up of department management, supervisors, and other key departmental personnel) to assist in the ongoing development of each department's implementation plan and to ensure a timely and thorough process.

Affiliating with Existing Programs

Many developing cardiovascular programs have benefited greatly from affiliating with other existing programs. Often this affiliation — generally between noncompeting hospitals — is simply an agreement on the part of the established program to provide information and education. The relationship may be the result of hospital ownership, as in the case of Catholic hospitals, or the result of a collegial relationship between participants, either members of the medical staffs or of the administration. Occasionally, a hospital looking to establish (or maintain) a relationship for the referral of difficult cases may extend this service to the new program; some hospitals will sell this service to developing programs.

Regardless of the arrangement, it is recommended that such affiliation be developed during implementation. This is because it is not always possible for the clinical team to gain its experience at the hospital where the cardiovascular surgeon will come from, although this is ideal.

Initiatives from large programs increasingly seek to formalize these relationships, thereby extending their market. Although no model has emerged yet, consideration should be given to a variety of alternative arrangements, including leasing facilities to the larger program or other joint venture relationships that allow for sharing risk and return. Such a linkage can not only reduce the risk from program start-up but also, in many situations, appease community concerns regarding the quality of a start-up program. This type of affiliation may also present patient service contracting opportunities in the managed care market that otherwise would be unavailable. Finally, an affiliation may provide access to clinicians and technicians (including nurses, anesthesiologists, perfusionists, surgeons, intensivists, pulmonologists, infectious disease physicians, and nephrologists) who are difficult to recruit and retain.

Summary

Planning a cardiovascular surgery program usually begins with hospital administrators responding to demand for more interventional cardiac facilities and should be a market-driven activity. Because cardiovascular surgical services will compete primarily on the basis of cost and quality—both determined by physicians' method of practice—surgeons must be recruited as early in the planning stage as possible. Standard recruitment incentives amy include guaranteed salary, start-up costs, and medical director pay.

Whether or not a cardiovascular surgeon has been selected by the time feasibility studies have given a proposed program the green light, a business plan must be written based on input from all departments that will be affected by the proposed cardiovascular surgery program. The business plan reflects three broad areas of agreement: It defines what is to be done, in what order, and during what time frame.

A formal business plan should have at least six sections that describe the project in more detail. The *executive summary* describes the scope of the CV surgery service—its objectives, resources required, and time frame for completion. The *program description* defines program components and other features. The *market analysis* highlights structures and characteristics of the market (referral patterns, demand projections). *Start-up* requirements list all resources (personnel, facilities, capital needs, physician referrals, and such) that are necessary to begin operations; this section also can be a basis for funding requests. *Marketing strategies* outline elements such as physician referral sources and practices, payer practices, and positioning of services in the market and how these will be used to compete in a market driven by physician referral. *Program management and organization* describes how implementation will be managed; it also describes organizational structure, reporting relationships, and what changes in structure may be needed after services are implemented. *Operations* will include an outline of how the new service will function—details will be developed during the implementation process. This section will also gauge whether new or added services can be delivered and caseload requirements (direct or indirect care) be fulfilled once services are added. Project phasing describes the order and timeline for implementation. Financial projections for five years should be included. A program evaluation mechanism should be developed and put into place.

A steering committee, the cardiovascular services planning committee (CSPC), is charged with implementation oversight and appointment of department task forces and subcommittees. Each task force will develop implementation plans and schedules from the perspective of individual departments that will be affected by the service addition; representatives from those departments will comprise task force membership. *All* departments (whether or not they are on a task force) should contribute to plan design and maintain an implementation program notebook describing how that department intends to prepare for the change in service (hiring or restructuring department personnel, for example).

Chapter 8

Strategic Marketing Plan

Competition among hospitals to attract patients, particularly cardiovascular patients, has become intense. In part this is due to the diversity of health care consumers — their number, their level of awareness of health care issues, and their purchasing power (from the single patient to bulk purchasers of health care services). As a result of these changes, hospitals must revise the way they manage this provider–consumer exchange.

Marketing is the management tool used to guide the interaction between service providers and their target markets. It must be used skillfully in developing and implementing cardiovascular programs and services, especially new ones. No longer is it adequate simply to plan and implement a new service or expand an existing one without giving careful attention to market factors. Planners and administrators must understand how market forces influence a consumer to choose one health care provider over another one.

Developing a carefully conceived, targeted marketing plan will help ensure that hospital resources are well spent. *Strategic marketing* is that portion of the marketing effort used in the development of strategies designed to ensure the successful attainment of specified objectives; it is the foundation of the marketing plan. This chapter discusses the strategic marketing plan and related process for cardiovascular programs and services. In addition, the concept of positioning will be discussed as a critical adjunct to marketing cardiovascular programs.

Developing the Marketing Plan

The marketing plan is an integrated document intended to guide the activities of a variety of participants to ensure that the marketing program is cohesive, thorough, timely, and efficient in its use of resources. Appendix D provides a sample outline of a strategic marketing plan for cardiovascular services.

In general, it is most effective to develop the plan with a small core group of individuals who will have the most input to the plan and subsequently will be held accountable for its implementation. Typically, this consists of the planning and marketing staff, the cardiovascular services manager/product line manager, the medical director, and selected others. The core group can be expanded on an ad hoc basis to develop or debate specific issues or segments of the plan. For example, if managed care is a key marketing target, patient services contracting should be dealt with extensively in the marketing plan; this will require input from the contracting staff.

Strategic market plans can be tailored to a specific service being implemented or expanded or to an entire program. For example, adding a new service (such as cholesterol screening) to an existing cardiovascular program will be fundamentally different from seeking increased utilization or increased patient volume for an existing service and therefore will require different plans. More complex cardiovascular programs—those that carry more economic and political risk or those facing existing or potential competition—will require more resources committed to marketing (particularly time and money).

It is recommended that a lead time of at least two years be allowed between plan development and implementation. This is because planning, construction, and approval can be lengthy processes and because virtually all marketing activities (from addition of new service announcements to collateral materials associated with patient services contracting) must be accounted for in the plan.

Like the business plan and the financial management plan, the marketing plan must be flexible enough to allow for changing circumstances that in turn will affect the plan and its timing. For example, launching a cardiac rehabilitation program will require different resources (and thus different timing parameters) than will initiating a cardiovascular surgery program.

Setting Out the Planning Process

Figure 8-1 displays a process for developing a strategic marketing plan that specifies the staff work and inputs needed so that management can make the decisions required to execute the plan.

Survey of Constituents

The first task in putting this process together is to survey program constituents—medical staff, board members, administrators, program physicians,

Figure 8-1. Strategic Marketing Planning Process

Staff Work and Inputs

Market Planning Outputs

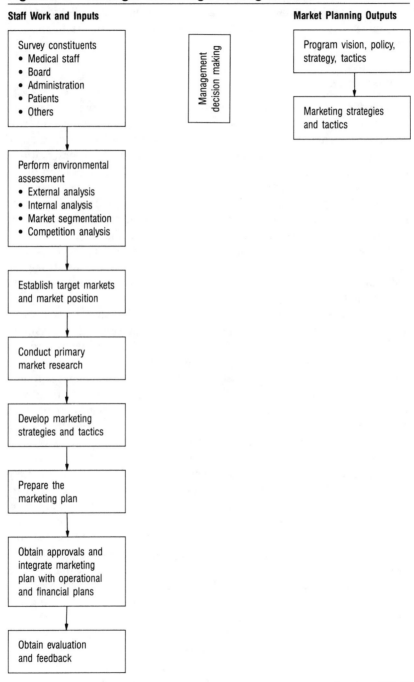

patients, major payers, and so forth. From this input, management constructs a vision. As detailed in chapter 4, this vision is expanded to include program policies, strategies, and tactics. This step forms the foundation for the plan.

Environmental Assessment

As noted in chapter 3, market assessment is the preliminary step in preparing a strategic marketing plan. This involves analyzing the internal and external environments, identifying the target markets and their needs, and identifying and examining the competition. From these observations, appropriate positioning for the service is determined. This portion of the process is most commonly referred to as the *environmental assessment.*

Upon completion, environmental assessment results are combined with the program vision to identify target markets and then prepare positioning statements for those target markets. As discussed in chapter 2, *positioning* is the attempt to differentiate among competing cardiovascular services along real dimensions — patient mix, average length of stay, medical staff credentials, and such — to ensure that the program or service is the right one for the targeted market segment(s).

Positioning relies largely on what phase of its life cycle a cardiovascular service is in (this is particularly true for cardiovascular surgery). For example, to position its service optimally one hospital might attempt either to introduce new services to the marketplace or to market services it already provides to new markets and/or new market segments. Another hospital might introduce services that, although new to that facility, are already available in the marketplace. In the latter situation, if the market is in its mature phase, then emphasizing how a service differs from existing services becomes the key positioning strategy and serves as the fulcrum for marketing campaigns.

As environments (both external and internal) continue to change, services must remain responsive and, therefore, be *repositioned* appropriately.

In promoting cardiovascular services, hospitals usually position themselves as technology leaders — depending on the range of services provided. For instance, community hospitals that provide "only" basic services usually do not compete on the basis of these services but on the basis that they provide cardiovascular surgery. This way they can promote their unique technology, high case volume, and thus their unique position in the marketplace.

Historically, the hospitals that provided cardiovascular surgery were large tertiary centers that commanded large market areas. However, over the past decade the proliferation of cardiovascular surgery programs into smaller community hospitals has diluted the market share of these former leaders. This market shift makes positioning a critical issue for *all* cardiovascular programs. Furthermore, it increases the importance of positioning a program or service that is effective *and* supported by market research.

Figure 8-2 is a list of potential differentiation strategies for cardiovascular services. Potential differentiation points are arrayed by marketing mix (product/service, price, promotion, and place/distribution). Each potential strategy needs to be weighed against the needs of the target market and balanced against program goals and objectives, as well as the overall positioning of the hospital in the community. Factors important to one or more significant target groups need to be considered as potential points of difference. For example, if a hospital directs its efforts to physicians, patients, and payers (three of the primary target groups) and if quality, price, and access are equally important differentiating factors to all three groups, then those factors could serve as the basis for the positioning strategy for all three target subsets.

Figure 8-2. Differentiation Strategies: Cardiovascular Services

Marketing Mix	Differentiation Points	
Product/service	• Pediatric surgery • Star-quality surgeon and/or cardiologist • Documentable quality • Program takes all comers —Clinically —Financially • Linkages/affiliations with more comprehensive programs • Preferred provider for many payers • Designation as center of excellence or institute of quality by major payer(s) • High volume relative to market	• Presence of research, unusual techniques, or high technology • Comprehensive array of diagnostic and therapeutic services • Chest pain emergency program • Heart institute • Teaching affiliation • Participation in cardiac emergency network • Electrophysiology services • Wellness and health promotion programs • Patient screening programs • Transplant • Laser capability
Price	• Low-price leader • Value leader (price and quality) • Total package price (hospital, surgeon, anesthesia, cardiologist, etc.)	• Participation in specialty PPO • Variable pricing
Promotion	• Physician referral system • Educational programs for target markets —Patients/consumers —Business/industry	• Physician network • Sales force for CV-related health, wellness, and educational programs to business/industry
Place/distribution	• Physical geographic location—accessibility to major markets • Convenience/patient orientation	• Satellite facilities • Cardiac emergency network • Mobile diagnostic services

Figure 8-3 lists typical information required to carry out the marketing plan. This information will vary considerably from place to place.

External Analysis

The external analysis should include an observation of the major trends and issues facing the health care marketplace that relate specifically to the hospital and its cardiovascular planning. Examples are the speed with which technology (such as laser angioplasty) is changing and changes in the underlying delivery system. Also, a shift in requirements for surgical backup for cardiac catheterization and other interventional procedures could have a tremendous impact on a program, as could the emergence of a medical group that combines large numbers of cardiovascular physicians.

Figure 8-3. Typical Data Requirements for a Cardiovascular Marketing Plan

- Historical definition of market area and appropriate listing of zip codes, with maps or charts if possible. Market area should be for cardiovascular patients (if existing service); or if data not available, for all hospital patients.
- Population and demographic analysis for defined market areas.
- Copy of hospital mission statement.
- Market share information—specific to cardiovascular patients and/or general hospital patients.
- Comparative utilization statistics on hospital and major competitors including figures such as number of open-heart surgeries, cardiac catheterizations, PTCAs, and so forth.
- All current promotional materials (samples) including collateral materials, advertisements, brochures, patient educational materials, symposium flyers, and such for the hospital as a whole and for cardiovascular activities in particular.
- Comparable promotional materials from hospital competitors.
- Competitor information—information on competitors, particularly those providing comparable levels of cardiovascular services.
- Copy of hospital overall strategic plan and/or marketing plan or pertinent portions thereof.
- Feasibility studies and/or business plans for cardiovascular services, as applicable.
- Consumer, payer, or physician primary market research reports conducted in the past 18 to 24 months.
- Copies of current patient satisfaction survey instruments and summary results for hospital and/or nursing units or for service elements specific to cardiovascular program.
- Managed care contracts and experience, including the following items:
  —List of contracts and performance information per contract, including parameters of contract, performance, and impact on hospital.
  —Contracts held by competitor hospitals.
  —List of top employers in the market area.
  —List of top payers in the market area.
- List of comparative pricing by targeted procedure for the market area, by major competitor and typical area contractual allowances. Include sample bills from other hospitals if possible.
- Available quality documentation on hospital and major competitors, such as published HCFA Medicare mortality data.
- Available information (objective or subjective) on competing physicians, including cardiovascular surgeons and cardiologists.

The external analysis will also identify and profile competitors and primary target groups (patients, payers, and physicians). (See chapter 3 for a discussion of gathering external data.)

Internal Analysis

Although critical to the success of the marketing plan, an understanding of the external environment must be balanced with a thorough grasp of the hospital's internal environment. One of the primary goals of an environmental assessment is to identify competitors, their strengths and weaknesses, and to predict their likely competitive actions and reactions. Internal analysis of the planning hospital along these same parameters must be performed to ensure a thorough understanding of the environment.

As a rule, the internal analysis portion of the strategic marketing plan will focus on the hospital's historical and ongoing activities that will support its entry into the market for cardiovascular services. Information should be gathered on utilization by type of service, payer class, profitability by program or service, physician activity indicators, physician resource consumption indicators, case cost data, and length of stay trends. Data should also be accumulated on DRGs and major inpatient and outpatient procedures.

The internal analysis should also ascertain facility design, equipment, and staffing strengths and weaknesses and how these will be influenced by new or expanded cardiovascular services. For example, if hospital A is adding a catheterization laboratory in remodeled space and hospital B recently added a similar laboratory in newly constructed space, hospital B may have a marketing advantage with physicians. If this is the case, then hospital A must develop marketing counterstrategies.

Other internal issues may be political, such as the degree of support or acceptability shown toward the cardiovascular service by current medical staff. Conflict within the medical community is not uncommon; for example, rarely is the cardiology staff perfectly situated or completely satisfied. Understanding the nature and intensity of the discontent can be beneficial; perhaps the problem is mandatory staff participation on the emergency room call panel or on the noninvasive interpretation panel. Changes to these policies can then be considered.

Market Segmentation

A critical portion of the plan requires segmenting the market, analyzing these segments, and targeting appropriate markets. The primary task of market segmentation involves dividing the market into smaller groups in order to understand more clearly their motivations, preferences, wants and needs. Figure 8-4 lists common major market segments and submarkets for cardiovascular services.

As always, because they control the referrals, physicians make up the most important segment for a subspecialty program. Within this segment are smaller segments that include referring cardiologists, primary care physicians, and medical groups.

Another principal segment comprises patients, who can be subdivided into smaller segments — former patients, cardiac patients, and female patients, for example. Other primary segments include business and industrial employers, governmental payers, private payers, and potential donors.

As target groups are better understood, marketing efforts can be customized even more to accommodate specific groups and attain more successful outcomes for the resources invested. Figure 8-5 shows criteria that various segmented and targeted markets could use in selecting a cardiovascular program. Each criterion is rated in importance — high, medium, and low. Ranking the importance of these criteria for each market segment helps identify the program elements that need the most attention and most immediate development throughout the marketing process.

The sample criteria in figure 8-5 can be estimated initially based on informal knowledge and common sense; primary market research and firsthand knowledge will further validate these base data. Managed care is an example of a force whose strength varies from community to community; where it is not a major force the cost and price criteria diminish in importance.

If discrepancies exist between what the market demands and what the program offers (or plans to offer), the organization must adjust plan development to align the two. For example, if the market demands a low price, the organization must first determine what "low price" means in the market, identify which market segments will respond at the target price, and develop a plan to deliver the service to the market at that target price.

Analysis of Competition

Every health care provider, regardless of mission, size, or ownership, must contend with actual or potential competition as a consequence of today's

Figure 8-4. Major Market Segments and Submarkets

- Physicians
  —Referring cardiologists
  —Primary care physicians
  —Medical groups
- Patients
  —Cardiac patients
  —Female patients
- Employers
  —Business/industry

- Governmental payers
  (Medicare, MediCal, other)
- Private payers (insurance companies, employers, health maintenance organizations, direct/self-pay, charity/free care)
- Potential donors

Figure 8-5. Major Markets and Identification of Program Selection Criteria

Criteria	Physicians			Patients			Industry			Payers			Donors			Employees		
	H	M	L	H	M	L	H	M	L	H	M	L	H	M	L	H	M	L
Cost/price	X				X		X			X				X				X
Location/convenience	X			X				X			X		X			X		
Interpersonal relations		X		X					X			X	X			X		
Modern facility/equipment	X			X				X			X		X			X		
High technology	X			X				X			X		X			X		
Facility ambience		X		X					X			X	X			X		
Waiting time	X			X					X			X			X	X		
Patient processing	X			X				X			X				X	X		
Overall quality reputation	X			X			X			X			X			X		
Exclusive contracting		X				X	X			X					X		X	
Proximity to hospital	X			X				X			X		X			X		
Recognition/feedback	X				X			X			X		X			X		

complex environment. Competition has transformed strategic formulation, planning, and marketing from theoretical concepts into mandatory behaviors. Strategy and ongoing operations will reflect other considerations to be sure, but the role of competition as an input will always be significant and increase in direct relation to its impact on the provider.

Because each state gathers hospital and physician data differently, the extent of the competitor data that can be gathered will vary substantially. Information available from the Health Care Financing Administration (HCFA) is generally too old, too cumbersome, or too limited to be used for competitive purposes. However, data bases are improving regularly; program administrators must stay abreast of the types and sources of data available within their states.

Primary Market Research

After service implementation, primary market research (community surveys or focus groups) may be needed to address unanswered questions for specific target markets and/or to serve as a baseline for measuring the effectiveness of marketing expenditure. This research may involve physicians, prospective patients, and payer markets in that all three have different opinions, attitudes, and priorities.

Typical market research questions include the following:

- What facility/sponsor is recognized by the surveyed population (patients, general population, employers, physicians, and so forth) as the leader in the service/program being studied? Why?
- What service attributes are important in selection of a program/service of this type? Price, availability/access, quality, others?
- How do patients access these services/programs? Physician referral, self-referral, combinations?
- How price-sensitive is the service/program?

Because primary market research is often an additional expense and may involve an outside vendor, it must be planned carefully and integrated into the planning process as early as possible.

Marketing Strategies and Tactics

Once constituents have been surveyed, an environmental assessment performed, targets and positions established, and primary research conducted, the *action* phase begins. This phase consists of strategy formulation and the development of marketing goals, tactics, or objectives. *All objectives must be strategically linked and support overall corporate objectives.*

As mentioned, marketing *strategies* outline a broad plan of action for using the hospital's resources to achieve a marketing goal or objective. Strategies themselves are the specific actions taken by the hospital to communicate with its target groups. Marketing *tactics* are specific plans of action that further define marketing strategies. Analogous to objectives, marketing tactics present basic objectives in more detail. Strategies and tactics can be developed and categorized into the conventional four *P*s of marketing (product, price, place, and promotion).

Goals are broad, unmeasurable statements with no time constraints. The following list is a representative sampling of goals developed for a new cardiovascular surgery and catheterization program (remember that *they are examples only*):

- Establish Memorial General Hospital and its physicians as leaders in the provision of comprehensive and innovative cardiovascular services in the South.
- Establish a partnership with physicians to support the development of comprehensive and innovative cardiovascular services.
- Provide state-of-the-art technology.
- Achieve superior clinical results and document quality outcomes over time.
- Compete successfully on "value"—the combined perceptions of quality and price—and continue to develop appropriate programs and methodologies to reduce the hospital's average cost per case while documenting clinical quality.
- Achieve budgeted levels of market share for cardiac surgery, catheterization, and coronary angioplasty and increase that market share over time.
- Provide a high level of customer satisfaction, based on customer wants and needs documented through market research.

After goals have been established, specific *objectives* need to be set. Objectives should cover important issues such as patient recognition or acceptability, physician utilization, and financial performance. Here is a representative sampling of objectives developed from the sample goals:

- Obtain target levels of cardiovascular service utilization of 40 cardiovascular surgeries, 90 cardiac catheterizations, and 30 PTCAs per month.
- Obtain a 35 percent rate of outpatient cardiac catheterization by the end of the first year of operation and incremental increases of 2.5 percent in subsequent years.
- Obtain an increase in level of customer awareness of the cardiovascular services at Memorial General Hospital of at least 10 percent by January 1993 (based on a baseline established in January 1991).

- Achieve an operational break-even financial position for the cardiac catheterization program by the end of the second year of operation.

Once goals and objectives have been set, it is necessary to "operationalize" them as specific tasks or tactics. Figure 8-6 includes some examples of strategies and tactics developed for a newly implemented cardiovascular surgery program in a competitive urban environment. Note that several tactics have been offered for each category of strategy—service (product), physical distribution (place), pricing, and promotion. This is important in that marketing is too frequently associated with advertising and promotion, which are only a portion of the overall marketing activities.

Marketing Plan Preparation

Final preparation of the plan is principally a matter of documentation and implementation. Organizational and staffing implications of the strategies and tactics may be outlined, including requirements for added staff necessary to fulfill proposed strategies and tactics or use of outside consultants, plus an appropriate organizational structure to accommodate staffing requirements.

All strategies and tactics have resource requirement implications, whether costs are direct or indirect. Planners must consider the cost of alternative strategies and tactics, and the expected return for each, as they are developed and debated among the work group. In addition, any budgetary constraints should be identified as early in the process as possible, because they will have a material impact on marketing strategies and tactics.

Integration of Marketing, Operational, Financial, and Human Resource Plans

Any strategic marketing plan must be integrated into the hospital's operational, financial, and human resource plans. Primarily this integration is to ensure that the financial resources required for plan implementation will be forthcoming and that the requisite political support is in place.

Each organization will incorporate into the approval and support processes administrative, medical staff, and board-level "sign off." Changes may be needed, and different resource levels may be required based on this approval process.

Evaluation and Feedback

Once the implementation is under way, a monitoring and reporting system will be necessary to evaluate the plan, tasks, and resources. Monitoring requires systematic periodic review of progress in each of these areas and

Figure 8-6. Sample Strategies and Tactics for a Cardiovascular Surgery Program

Service Strategies

1. In all marketing communications with each target public, communicate the differential advantages of CV surgery at XYZ Medical Center:
   - Star-quality surgeon
   - Demonstrable quality based on track record of surgeon and team
   - Comparable home service provided locally and conveniently to patients
2. Emphasize the concept of personal service, patient-friendly systems, and high-quality management as basis of relationship between XYZ Medical Center and its patients.
3. Design and implement a formal policy, procedure, and process to monitor cardiovascular surgery patient satisfaction.
   - Develop a brief patient satisfaction survey form to be administered by a "neutral" party.
   - Survey 100 percent of all CV surgery patients during first year of operation to ascertain their level of satisfaction.
   - Analyze all results from the patient satisfaction surveys, making appropriate system and other changes to increase level of satisfaction.
   - After the first year of operation, survey an appropriate percentage of CV patients on a predetermined, periodic, in-depth basis to ascertain level of satisfaction.

Physical Distribution Strategies

1. In all marketing communications with each target market, communicate the differential advantages of CV surgery at XYZ Medical Center, including comparable home services provided conveniently to patient.
2. A "push" in direct distribution strategy will be developed to capitalize on the loyalty among actual and potential referring cardiologists in the greater _____ area.
3. A "pull" in direct distribution strategy will be developed to create a preference for XYZ Medical Center among potential patients requiring CV surgery. However, it is required that patient preferences be cultivated/managed over time so that patients directed to XYZ Medical Center will see this choice as logical, offering decided benefits, and of comparable quality.

Pricing Strategies

1. A pricing strategy should be set for CV surgery retail prices at current market rates for the first 150 cases or until procedural/case experience or financial analysis indicates otherwise. It is believed that PPO contracts will be generally unavailable until XYZ Medical Center completes 150 cases.
   - Retail price should be based on a detailed line item bill analysis from a representative sample of cases at ABC Medical Center.
   - Because retail patients do not respond to price reductions, consideration will be given to increasing certain surgical charges or to adding new chargeable items in order to maintain a reasonable retail price.
     —Retail price less a cash discount will be given to international Asian patients.
   - Because it is assumed that 70 percent of CV patients will be Medicare insured, it will be important to set retail prices and control costs to maximize the margin.
2. Managed care prices (HMO/PPO) should be set in anticipation of the availability of contracts and/or the completion of 150 surgical cases. Case prices should be based on comparable case rates in the market area.

(Continued on next page)

Figure 8-6. (Continued)

Promotion Strategies

1. Create an awareness campaign designed to communicate the establishment and implementation of the CV surgery program to target markets, using standard public relations methods and activities. For example:
   • Press releases and dissemination of press kits
   • Cardiac pavilion physician open house
   • Cardiac pavilion community open house and health fair
   • Personal or other communications to donor groups
   • Stories in appropriate internal communications for employees, volunteers, and so forth
   • Presentations by administration to employees, volunteers, donor groups, and so forth
2. Create an awareness campaign designed to communicate the establishment of the CV surgery program to current and potential referring physicians. For example:
   • A personal letter from Dr. _____ to his past referral sources in the greater _____ area informing them that his services will be available at XYZ Medical Center, along with pertinent other details of the program
   • A letter from XYZ Medical Center and/or Dr. _____ to potential referring physicians encouraging their participation
   • Appropriate informational pieces placed in the medical staff bulletin or communicated in other ways to current staff physicians
3. Design and develop marketing communications materials to include the following:
   • A program name and logo
   • A patient teaching package, including comprehensive materials for presurgical and postsurgical patient education
   • A cardiovascular services general brochure to be direct mailed
   • Referring physician package including overview of program, information for physician referral, patient follow-up, etc.
   • Patient brochures (in the following priority/budget order):
     —Cardiovascular surgery
     —Cardiac catheterization
     —PTCA
     —Cardiac rehabilitation
   • A managed care package to include the above-referenced materials plus information specific to payers/purchasers

---

a mechanism for adopting inevitable changes. The cardiovascular administrator must work with the planning and marketing staff in evaluating results, and all findings must be reported to program constituents through regular channels.

Anticipating Problems and Limitations of the Marketing Plan

The mere existence of a marketing plan — no matter how well conceived and executed — will not ensure the financial and operational success of a cardiovascular program or service. Potential problems and pitfalls include the following:

- No amount of marketing effort can salvage a poorly designed program.
- Failure to evaluate the marketplace objectively can lead to too much "inside out" marketing. Effective market research precludes this.
- Failure to identify and analyze target groups will cripple a plan.
- Failure to involve physicians appropriately in the process can lead to underestimating or overestimating the effect of self-referrals and relying too heavily on advertising and promotion for a program not heavily influenced by self-referrals.
- Failure to provide adequate financial resources to achieve stated goals and objectives will undermine a program.
- Failure to assign task responsibility and monitor results can lead to an inability to adequately evaluate customer satisfaction.

It cannot be overemphasized that marketing is political in nature and can upset the political balance of physician referral patterns and other "natural" balances within the community. Therefore, it is incumbent on every individual involved in the marketing effort to be sensitive to political realities and to develop activities that build on natural alliances and mutual benefits.

Summary

Strategic marketing plans should be developed for all cardiovascular service offerings, whether new or current. Effective planning relies on having a thorough understanding of internal and external hospital environments. Two key factors, identifying and analyzing target markets *and* positioning the service offering within the competitive environment, should underlie the marketing plan. Analysis should also include studying the competition, evaluating strengths and weaknesses, considering factors internal to the hospital, and considering the product life cycle phase of the proposed offering and any competing offerings. Primary market research (focus groups, questionnaires, surveys) may be needed to ascertain answers that cannot be arrived at through secondary means. Once all analyses are complete, the action phase begins, which includes drafting goals, objectives, strategies, and tactics and matching them with appropriate levels of resource requirements.

After the implementation of the marketing plan begins, a monitoring and reporting system must be in place to effectively evaluate results and provide accurate information with which to guide the refinement of the effort.

Chapter 9

Diagnostic and Therapeutic Cardiovascular Technology

Contemporary diagnosis and treatment of cardiovascular disease has become technology intensive and technology dependent. This chapter describes the various diagnostic and therapeutic modalities conventionally applied in cardiovascular services. This chapter is organized into five sections:

1. Noninvasive cardiology diagnostic modalities
2. Invasive cardiology diagnostic procedures
3. Therapeutic or interventional invasive cardiology procedures
4. Cardiac surgery interventions
5. Recent developments and ongoing research

Cardiovascular therapy, whether medical or procedural, initially is based on noninvasive diagnostic studies. Noninvasive procedures can be as simple as the basic 12-lead electrocardiogram (EKG) or as complex as the recently introduced transesophageal echocardiogram (TEE).

Many patients undergo much of this testing (including the most sophisticated procedures) as outpatients at their cardiologist's office. Others receive in-hospital testing either as outpatients or inpatients. As a result of the proliferation of diagnostic equipment into physicians' offices, some hospital cardiology departments are in direct competition with local cardiologists for patients for these procedures. In many cases the local cardiologist is also the department's medical director, thereby complicating the competitive nature of the hospital–physician relationship. Learning to recognize and manage this competition is a key strategy for hospitals in developing new alliances with cardiologists or strengthening existing ones. Many successful hospital-based noninvasive cardiology services seek to provide the full spectrum of diagnostic procedures for the hospital's general medical staff patients while working with competing cardiologists to identify the most sophisticated (and generally most expensive) technology to offer as adjuncts to what is offered in the physicians' offices.

The decision on which diagnostic procedure to use generally depends on the diagnostic information the physician is searching for, but sometimes more than one modality can be used to gather similar information. Where appropriate, this chapter will indicate these crossover modalities and their competitive technologies.

Noninvasive Cardiology Diagnostic Modalities

Noninvasive diagnostic cardiology experienced significant growth during the 1970s and 1980s. The addition of cardiac ultrasound (echocardiography/cardiac Doppler) as well as nuclear cardiology was primarily responsible for this growth. Ongoing improvements in accuracy and reliability have contributed to the proliferation of these modalities throughout the health care delivery system.

A comprehensive noninvasive cardiology program provides several specialized procedures. In that this book focuses on cardiology programs, it will not cover noninvasive vascular technology. Although many cardiology departments provide these services, they generally do so under the associated title of noninvasive vascular laboratory services.

The following sections describe procedures provided by comprehensive noninvasive diagnostic cardiology departments.

Electrocardiography

Electrocardiography is the recording and study of electrocardiograms (graphic records) of the electrical signals originating from the heart. The electrocardiogram, typically referred to as ECG or EKG, is used routinely as a diagnostic test for cardiac disease. Popular variations of the EKG (discussed in subsequent sections) are the stress EKG and ambulatory EKG recording (Holter monitoring). Another specialized form of electrocardiographic recording is the permanent pacemaker analysis recording. These procedures are individually described in sections to follow.

Used nearly as often as routine blood tests and chest X-rays, the EKG provides the physician with considerable information relating to the patient's current or prior cardiac status. Common diagnostic reasons for performing an electrocardiogram include the need to assess cardiac rhythm and rate, to look for indications of reduced blood flow to the heart (known as cardiac ischemia), and to detect evidence of previous heart attack or impending heart attack (myocardial infarction, or MI).

The routine EKG is provided in all hospitals and most physicians' offices through the use of electrocardiographic recorders. A typical EKG recorder is mounted on a mobile pedestal for ease in moving it to the patient's bedside.

Currently, these recording devices are available with on-board, computerized interpretation capabilities. Computer-interpreted EKGs have become increasingly more common in many hospitals as the interpretation programs have become more accurate and sophisticated. The computer-interpreted EKG provides the primary care physician with an interim confirmation of EKG diagnoses that will be monitored by the specialist for computer accuracy.

Historically, many physicians have opposed this computer-assisted technology, but as the interpretation programs have improved in accuracy many now find this "unverified" reporting to be acceptable. Most (if not all) hospitals with computerized EKG interpretation equipment require that these reports be "overread" (monitored) by the staff physician, as with non–computer-interpreted EKGs.

The computer-interpreted EKG market has provided an offshoot technology as well. To prepare an EKG for computer interpretation, the EKG recorder must convert the patient's EKG waveforms into digitized information. In response, EKG equipment manufacturers have developed computer-based EKG record storage systems for hospitals and medical offices. Once used only by large tertiary medical centers, EKG storage computer systems are now available based on personal computer (PC) technology at significantly reduced and affordable prices. The latest generation of EKG recorders are smaller and provide extensive operator amenities that enhance accuracy and productivity. This trend will probably continue.

The other major change in EKG service in recent years has been the further development of computer-interpreted systems and computer storage systems. Ongoing improvement in computerized interpretation programs is expected to continue as providers of equipment compete in this marketplace. Reliability of equipment and accuracy of interpretation programs will be the standards for competition, with increasing emphasis on centralized, computer-based record storage systems.

In their efforts to improve cardiology department productivity, many hospitals will look to investing in EKG record storage computer systems that will also allow storage of Holter records, stress EKG tracings, and word-processed reports for all records produced in their department. No other significant changes in EKG technology are expected in the near future.

Stress Electrocardiography

Although informative and cost-effective to administer, the EKG is limited in the scope of diagnostic data it can provide. These limitations are due mainly to the short duration of time (10–12 seconds) over which an EKG records the patient's heart rhythm. To enhance the effectiveness of electrocardiography as a "predictor" of future cardiac episodes, such as heart attacks, methods have been developed that incorporate modified forms of EKG recording. Stress electrocardiography is one of these modifications.

The main purpose of this procedure (commonly called treadmill testing) is to examine the patient's EKG, blood pressure, and other information about the patient's cardiac status *during exercise* to help determine whether the patient has significant coronary artery disease (arterial lesions). The patient is connected to an electrocardiograph, and recordings of EKG and blood pressure are made before, during, and after exercising on a treadmill device. In an effort to condense the work load or physical stress that the patient experiences, the treadmill is capable of changing speed (by accelerating or reducing belt action) and elevation (angle of incline) in precise increments.

The principle behind the procedure is that if the patient's blood flow is restricted by lesions in the coronary artery system, certain changes should occur in the EKG or blood pressure response if the patient exercises to a point where the heart muscle requires more blood than the obstructed artery can provide.

This procedure can be performed in a number of variations that allow the physician to test for more specific purposes or to enhance the inherent accuracy of the procedure. These alternative stress test procedures include:

- Low-level stress testing (post-MI patients and patients with reduced physical tolerance)
- Nuclear cardiography procedures (stress thallium or stress multiple-gated acquisition — MuGA)
- Stress echocardiography

The basic equipment required for stress testing includes an EKG recorder and monitor (preferably with three channels) to visualize the patient's EKG at all times during exercise and a blood pressure manometer and cuff. An emergency cart (crash cart) should also be made available in case problems arise during the procedure (problems can range in severity from slight difficulty in breathing to fatal heart attack). The emergency cart should store a range of equipment: medications, intravenous fluids and administration sets, syringes and needles, oxygen (either in a portable bottle or from a wall-mounted source with associated delivery equipment), intubation supplies and equipment, and a suction unit with catheters.

Although actual performance of stress EKG procedures requires no extensive training, the possibility of medical complications requires that assisting personnel be trained in emergency medical procedures. A minimum level of emergency procedure competence is completion of the American

Heart Association basic cardiac life support (BCLS) module. Personnel trained in advanced cardiac life support (ACLS) are desirable; these personnel may be the hospital's "code blue" team.

Depending on the equipment being used or the condition of the patient being stressed, one or two staff members may be required to perform stress EKG procedures. A stress EKG laboratory (or lab room) should be large enough to accommodate the patient, staff, and equipment, including the emergency cart, oxygen, and the patient's bed.

Stress EKG technology is not expected to change significantly in the short-term future. It will, however, continue to experience competition from new technologies. Many physicians do not consider standard stress electrocardiography to be sensitive enough in detecting the existence of significant coronary artery disease. The accurate, noninvasive detection of coronary artery disease is the focus of researchers worldwide; consequently, several alternative procedures have been developed or are under development. Currently, stress echocardiography and nuclear cardiography procedures compete for this segment of patients. The competitive procedures of the future are expected to include cine computed tomography (CT), high-speed magnetic resonance imaging (MRI), and positron emission tomography (PET), which are reported to assess noninvasively the patient's myocardial perfusion (flow of oxygenated blood to and through the heart muscle).

Ambulatory EKG Recording

To assess cardiac rhythm for a longer period of time (the electrical signal that controls the heart's activity), the physician uses ambulatory EKG recording, also called Holter monitoring. A monitoring device is connected to the patient to record cardiac rhythm (EKG signal) for 24 hours or longer while a computer system analyzes all recorded beats.

The most commonly used system records two channels of the patient's EKG onto a cassette tape while the patient performs most normal functions, including exercise and other strenuous activities. The system incorporates a computerized analysis module, which allows the technologist to "scan" the 24 hours of recorded cardiac activity for abnormalities and generate a customized report. Usually a report can be generated in 45 to 60 minutes.

The fundamental purpose of this procedure is to allow the physician to evaluate a patient's EKG activity over an extended time to detect any abnormality. The physician may be diagnosing for symptoms of dizziness or fainting during activity or evaluating cardiac waveforms during exercise to determine whether there is evidence of coronary ischemia or insufficient blood supply to the heart. Used for inpatients and outpatients, ambulatory EKG monitoring in most settings generally is higher in volume for outpatients than for inpatients. This is because the test is considered highly accurate for assessing cardiac rhythm in normal life situations. The physical connection and removal of the recording device and the scanning of the recording comprise the bulk of the time necessary to process these procedures, with an average of 60 to 90 minutes of technician's time required per patient.

As in other EKG technology, the greatest changes in ambulatory EKG monitoring have been in the area of computer-assisted analysis of the recorded information. Strides in accuracy and speed have constituted the primary areas of competition among manufacturers, although some improvement has been noted in the reliability of the recording devices after manufacturers developed a digital recorder that stores EKG waveforms in computer memory. Most manufacturers have reduced the size of the recorders as well.

The improvements in diagnostic accuracy have increased the use of ambulatory EKG monitoring in the areas of silent myocardial ischemia and atrial arrhythmias. At this time, neither current nor future alternative technologies seem poised to enter the marketplace.

Cardiac Ultrasound (Echocardiography/Cardiac Doppler)

Cardiologists routinely use cardiac ultrasound imaging, known as echocardiography, to provide direct imaging of the heart and its associated structures. This ultrasound technique generates a highly accurate, cross-sectional image of the heart to visualize cardiac wall motion and valve function and to test for the presence of structural abnormalities for congenital heart disease.

As a subspecialty of ultrasonography, this completely noninvasive procedure has become a dominant tool over the past decade. Significant improvements in image resolution and development of related technologies (such as cardiac Doppler procedures) have catapulted echocardiography into its strong position in noninvasive diagnostic cardiology.

Doppler ultrasound was named after the Austrian physicist and mathematician Christian Johann Doppler, who discovered the physical principle called the Doppler effect. The Doppler effect is based on the fact that electromagnetic waves reflected from a body in motion change wavelength depending on whether the body is traveling away from or toward the point of observation. In Doppler ultrasound, a transducer is directed at a blood vessel or heart chamber, and sound waves are reflected off the red blood cells. If blood flow is toward the transducer, the wavelength is narrowed, and conversely, if the direction of flow is away from the transducer, the wavelength is widened. This information is then transformed into an audible sound signal and a graphic display for the technician and physician, who can then evaluate blood flow direction and velocity.

In addition to being highly useful for adult cardiology, echocardiography/cardiac Doppler has also become an indispensable tool of pediatric cardiologists in their evaluation of congenital heart disease patients. Many pediatric cardiologists have come to believe that echocardiography can be more valuable than cardiac catheterization in their diagnosis of certain congenital cardiac abnormalities. At many centers it has become routine to perform surgical corrections for certain congenital abnormalities on the basis of echo/Doppler findings alone.

The equipment used to perform these procedures consists of an ultrasound processing unit (the echocardiograph) and the handheld ultrasound generator–receiver unit known as the transducer. The echocardiograph generally is portable and can process, view, and record the ultrasound information that is generated. The ultrasound transducer connects to the echocardiograph so that the technologist can transmit and receive the ultrasound energy into and from the patient's heart. Ultrasound transducers are manufactured in various frequency ranges to provide optimal imaging capability for different patients, primarily according to the size of the patient. An echo laboratory that provides imaging services to all patients, adult and pediatric, will generally utilize up to four different frequencies of transducers.

Many hospitals have combined their echocardiography equipment and real-time ultrasound (usually radiology department–based) units by purchasing a single system, which has the capability to provide imaging and Doppler studies for cardiac imaging, noninvasive vascular evaluation, and abdominal ultrasound procedures. This combination of imaging modalities into one system can be a valuable method to upgrade a hospital's ultrasound capabilities — if no one area of need is exceptionally busy. However, this approach loses efficiency if any one department begins to need the system more frequently than other departments, causing scheduling conflicts. Most larger hospitals have invested in separate, dedicated systems for each area of ultrasound specialization.

The current generation of systems offers pulsed wave and continuous wave cardiac Doppler capability and now are standard with color-flow Doppler. A recognizable trend in cardiac ultrasound equipment is the built-in upgradability of each module of the system to minimize long-term obsolescence.

The following section describes echocardiography/cardiac Doppler procedures and how they are used in the diagnosis of cardiac disease.

M-Mode Echocardiography

Motion-mode (M-mode) echocardiography generally has been incorporated into the current standard procedure known as two-dimensional (2-D) echocardiography. Motion-mode echo provides the physician with a static, paper printout utilizing a linear representation of the motion of the cardiac structures. Motion-mode recordings provide the means to accurately measure cardiac chamber dimensions, heart wall thicknesses, and valve opening and velocity values.

Two-Dimensional Echocardiography

Two-dimensional echocardiography currently is the mainstay of this group of cardiac ultrasound modalities. As stated previously, 2-D echo provides the physician with accurate cross-sectional views of the heart and its related structures and vessels. These real-time images are used to evaluate the wall motion and chamber sizes of the heart.

Pulsed Wave and Continuous Wave Cardiac Doppler

Cardiac Doppler procedures permit the assessment of intracardiac blood flow, both qualitatively and quantitatively. Pulsed Doppler detects evidence of abnormal blood flow such as cardiac valvular regurgitation. Continuous wave cardiac Doppler evaluates blood flow velocity and volume. This technique is used noninvasively to estimate the severity of cardiac valvular stenosis (narrowing of the cardiac valve opening) or to assess the volume of blood that regurgitates through a leaking heart valve.

Color-Flow Cardiac Doppler

A relatively new cardiology procedure, color-flow Doppler provides a method to visualize intracardiac and extracardiac blood flow while simultaneously visualizing cardiac structures. This is achieved by superimposing a color image representation of the blood flow patterns over the standard black-and-white image of the cardiac structures in a 2-D process (in essence, color-flow Doppler can be considered a 2-D Doppler). The blood flow imaging and velocity analysis facilitated by these systems can be accomplished with considerably more ease and speed than conventional pulsed wave and continuous wave methods. Furthermore, this technique allows those new to Doppler technology to quickly orient themselves and learn the associated techniques more rapidly.

Color-flow Doppler provides diagnostic assistance to the cardiologist for many abnormal cardiac conditions. For example, cardiac valvular insufficiency or regurgitation is readily visualized with this technique, which can also supply information on the volume of regurgitant blood flow. Congenital cardiac defects are diagnosed more readily after intracardiac blood flow conditions are understood more clearly. This can be accomplished safely and noninvasively with echocardiography and color-flow Doppler in nearly all conditions.

Stress Echocardiography

Stress echocardiography combines the cardiac imaging capabilities of echocardiography and the electrocardiographic and blood pressure assessment of standard stress testing. The echo imaging component allows the physician to visualize the heart muscle (myocardium) during exercise to detect areas of reduced motion or contraction due to reduced blood supply. Reduced cardiac wall motion or contractility infers the presence of lesions that restrict blood flow in the coronary artery system responsible for blood supply to the affected area.

The noninvasive evaluation of coronary artery disease was accomplished in the past by using the treadmill stress test, with or without nuclear isotope imaging. This way, the physician had EKG and blood pressure recordings before, during, and after physically stressing the patient on a treadmill. This procedure was shown to have an overall accuracy of approximately 75 percent, increasing to 90 percent or higher with the addition of nuclear imaging.

Several studies have shown that by combining echo imaging of the heart during stress and the stress EKG and blood pressure data, highly accurate assessment for coronary artery disease can be achieved when the procedure is performed under well-controlled conditions. Many users of this technology believe that they are achieving more than 90 percent accuracy. Stress echocardiography requires a sophisticated microcomputer-based analysis system that assists with comparing images "at rest" and images "under stress." The cardiologist making the interpretation reviews these results to determine whether the heart muscle being imaged shows an inappropriate reduction of contraction during the exercise.

Intraoperative Cardiac Doppler (Echo/Doppler)

Some cardiac surgery facilities have begun to utilize echo/Doppler for perioperative and postsurgical evaluation of results. This technique originally involved direct imaging of the heart and its structures while the patient's chest was still open. This "open-chest" methodology essentially has been replaced with the transesophageal echo/Doppler modality described in the next section.

Transesophageal Echo/Doppler

Transesophageal echo/Doppler (TEE) requires a specialized transducer mounted on the end of an esophageal probe. By inserting this esophageal transducer into the patient's esophagus, the physician is able to obtain images of the heart and Doppler blood flow recordings taken in close proximity to the cardiac structures. This technique has been shown to significantly enhance the resolution of the images being visualized. Applications include the intraoperative monitoring of cardiac wall motion to detect early evidence of perioperative myocardial infarction and the postsurgical evaluation of cardiac valve replacement and other repair procedures. Additionally, TEE can be used to evaluate patients who cannot be imaged adequately by conventional methods.

Nuclear Imaging

The use of nuclear imaging techniques to diagnose cardiovascular disease became more commonplace during the 1980s. Two modalities predominate: stress EKG testing combined with thallium uptake scanning and technetium-gated blood pool studies (MuGA). Each of these nuclear scanning procedures may be done with the patient at rest, thus eliminating the stress EKG component.

Stress thallium testing is utilized to increase the accuracy of the standard stress EKG procedure in the detection of coronary artery disease. The radioisotope is injected at or near the peak point of exercise and circulates through the patient's tissues, being absorbed in higher quantities by oxygenated cardiac muscle tissue. After the exercise is finished, the patient is scanned by a computer-assisted nuclear scintillation camera to image and record the cardiac muscle for areas of reduced uptake of the isotope. This procedure, when performed under optimal conditions, has been shown to be very accurate for coronary artery disease detection.

Technetium cardiac studies, or MuGA (multiple-gated acquisition), scans use a different isotope that tags to the patient's red blood cells, allowing scintillation camera imaging of the larger areas of blood pools within the body. The most common procedure using this isotope is the stress MuGA exam that analyzes cardiac wall motion during stress exercise to detect evidence of coronary artery disease. If the patient's coronary arterial system is significantly obstructed, abnormal cardiac wall motion changes will occur during exercise.

Recently, single-photon emission computerized tomography (SPECT) has enhanced nuclear cardiology imaging capability through improved imaging resolution and reduced imaging times. This upgraded modality, which requires use of special nuclear imaging cameras combined with specially prepared radiopharmaceuticals, is the current standard for nuclear cardiac imaging. Many physicians believe that SPECT imaging, combined with ECG stress testing, is the most accurate noninvasive diagnostic technique for coronary artery disease.

Invasive Cardiology Procedures

In the past, invasive diagnostic cardiology procedures were required before patients could undergo corrective or palliative (reducing pain or other symptoms without curing) cardiac surgery. With the development of interventional (therapeutic) catheterization techniques, invasive cardiology has undergone a major change of focus and is now seen as the state-of-the-art treatment of choice for many patients. Specifically the change is due to evolution of percutaneous transluminal coronary angioplasty (PTCA), valvuloplasty, permanent pacemaker implantation, and therapeutic electrophysiology procedures to the point where they are routinely performed in cardiac catheterization laboratories nationwide.

The following section describes diagnostic and therapeutic invasive cardiology techniques, their applications in the diagnosis and treatment of cardiac disease, and information related to providing these services.

Diagnostic Cardiac Catheterization

Since the 1950s, cardiac catheterization procedures have become the definitive diagnostic tool for evaluation of most forms of cardiac disease (including congenital heart disease and valvular heart disease). Diagnostic cardiac catheterization is an X-ray (radiographic) technique. It uses various vascular catheters to deliver opaque contrast (iodine-based dye) injections into the cardiac chambers and/or coronary arteries and is coupled with high-speed, high-resolution, 35-mm filming capabilities of the images that are produced. The recording of intracardiac and intravascular pressures and the collection of blood samples for oxygen content analysis complete the information gathered during this invasive procedure.

Cardiac catheterization was initially used to diagnose congenital heart disease and to observe activity in the cardiac chambers and associated large vessels; this process was the angiography. A technique to view the arteries supplying the heart muscle tissue (nonselective coronary arteriography) was subsequently developed, followed by development of a technique to view specific coronary arteries (selective coronary arteriography). This latter technique provides significantly enhanced, high-resolution images of the coronary arteries and atherosclerotic lesions through use of specialized catheters designed to access the openings of each coronary artery. These catheterization procedures are named for the physicians who perfected them.

With the Judkins technique, the catheter is inserted percutaneously (needled puncture through the skin) into an artery in the groin and threaded retrograde to the opening of the coronary arteries and through the aortic valve into the left ventricle. The Sones technique requires the physician to surgically open the brachial artery in the arm or "cuts down" to access the arterial system.

A component of diagnostic cardiac catheterization is the recording and evaluation of the pressures within the cardiac chambers, pulmonary artery or arteries, pulmonary capillary vessels (after temporarily blocking forward flow with a balloon-tipped catheter to measure the back pressure from the left atrium), aorta, and venous vessels. Known as *hemodynamic monitoring and recording,* these pressure readings require the use of sensitive and accurate vascular pressure recording systems. When the recording of intra-vascular pressures is performed along with the recording of additional information, such as EKG signals, this is known as *physiologic monitoring and recording.*

Cardiac catheterization — particularly the advent of selective coronary arteriography and recordation of hemodynamic pressures — led directly to the development of coronary artery bypass graft (CABG) surgery in the 1960s. Reliable and consistently accurate diagnosis of coronary artery disease occlusions, along with the development of appropriate surgical techniques, gave surgeons the precision needed to graft (anastomose) a vessel to the proper points below the arterial lesion in order to bypass the blockage and restore near-normal blood flow to the heart.

Cardiac catheterization procedures require a specialized radiographic (X-ray) procedure room equipped with high-resolution, high-speed, 35-mm filming and videotaping capabilities. The cardiologist uses a high-resolution fluoroscopic (live X-ray) imaging system to visualize the catheter's position within the patient so as to position the catheter to perform the contrast injections required to visualize the cardiac chamber or vessel for filming or recording the intravascular pressure.

Many hospitals have a radiographic room dedicated as a cardiac catheterization laboratory. This allows lab equipment to be configured optimally for highest-quality images of cardiac structures and coronary arteries. By using a small-diameter image intensifier (II) of 7 to 9 inches, the laboratory can provide higher resolution for film and video recordings.

Another approach (used at many hospitals) is to combine a radiology department special procedures laboratory, also known as an angiographic suite, and a cardiac catheterization laboratory. Because each discipline provides angiograms as one of the end products — coronary angiography is essentially a specialized form of general angiography — this can be a natural solution for many hospitals. That is, by combining these services into one radiographic room the hospital saves the space and capital expenditure the other radiographic room would require. Sharing personnel and supplies can further reduce the cost of providing these services.

The downside to this combination approach is recurring scheduling conflicts between radiologists and cardiologists and the need for large-image intensifiers for radiographic procedures, which most likely will not provide optimal cardiac images. Many hospitals in overcoming these problems continue to provide cardiac catheterization services through the use of a modified special procedures radiographic room.

Other routine diagnostic cardiac catheterization procedures include the following:

- *Left-heart catheterization with selective coronary arteriography (occasionally requires right-heart catheterization) — adult:* The most common diagnostic cardiac catheterization procedure performed, this invasive test is used to image and film the patient's coronary arteries and left ventricle and to record intravascular pressures from the aorta and left ventricle. When the procedure is combined with a right-heart catheterization procedure, a record is made of intravascular pressures from the patient's right atrium, right ventricle, and pulmonary arteries, and both central venous blood samples and arterial blood samples are obtained for estimated cardiac output calculations.

- *Right-heart and/or left-heart catheterization for diagnosis of congenital heart disease — pediatric:* This technique is used to diagnose congenital cardiac disease and frequently requires cardiac chamber and great vessel angiography. Most common congenital defects of the heart involve abnormal openings of either the interatrial septum or the interventricular septum or abnormal communication channels between large vessels, such as *patent ductus arteriosus.* Other defects may involve abnormally developed cardiac valves, chambers, or restricted major vessels leaving the heart. The cardiologist will film various views of these abnormalities, record intracardiac and intravascular pressure waveforms, and collect blood samples to analyze the severity of the abnormality.

- *Right-heart catheterization to diagnose pulmonary disease including pulmonary angiography for pulmonary embolism — adult:* This procedure involves only the right-heart chambers and vessels. The cardiologist inserts a catheter into the patient's venous system only and manipulates the catheter through the right-heart chambers into the pulmonary artery. Angiography and pressure recordings are then performed to diagnose the extent of the patient's condition.

Electrophysiology

Electrophysiology (EP) is used to diagnose and locate regions of abnormal cardiac electrical signal formation (arrhythmogenesis). Multiple-electrode catheters are positioned in atria and/or ventricles to selectively stimulate an area of cardiac tissue so that the electrophysiologist can record the electrical signals generated from the patient's heart. A major use for EP is to assess the cardiac conduction system of a patient being considered for permanent pacemaker implantation so as to determine whether treatment should be medical therapy or therapeutic electrophysiology.

Electrophysiology is also used therapeutically, either in the catheterization laboratory or in the cardiac surgery suite. Therapeutic EP procedures performed in the catheterization laboratory use substantial quantities of electrical energy delivered to a select area of cardiac tissue. The high dosage causes that tissue to lose its electrical conductivity. This procedure is known as *catheter ablation.*

In the cardiac surgery suite EP is used to diagnose and locate myocardial tissue that will be surgically removed or cryogenically frozen (cryoablation). These procedures are performed to eliminate areas of injured heart tissue (usually from a myocardial infarction) that cause uncontrollable and life-threatening arrhythmias.

These procedures continue to be the highest quality of diagnostic tests for coronary artery disease and most other cardiac-related pathology. The steady increase of PTCA procedures throughout the country has increased the use of diagnostic cardiac catheterization as more physicians treat acute MI patients with thrombolytic agents to reverse the infarction process. This has resulted in patients' requiring invasive diagnostic studies to evaluate the severity of their coronary artery disease after their condition stabilizes.

As mentioned earlier, the utilization rate for diagnostic cardiac catheterization has steadily increased over the past several years and will most likely continue to do so for several more years. This trend is linked to an aging population and wider availability of catheterization procedures.

Other, less invasive procedures are being investigated to replace coronary angiography for the diagnosis of coronary artery disease. These include high-speed computed tomography (CT) and magnetic resonance imaging (MRI). To date, these modalities have not proved effective in providing the imaging resolution necessary to replace coronary arteriography.

Therapeutic or Interventional Invasive Procedures

Invasive cardiology procedures can be therapeutic or diagnostic. Therapeutic invasive procedures are also referred to as interventional. Interventional cardiology has undergone constant upgrading over the past decade to the point where it has revolutionized treatment of heart disease. For example, interventions such as PTCA, pacemaker implants, or ablation have made it possible for certain patients—those with coronary artery disease, cardiac valvular disease, or congenital heart disease—to be treated by cardiologists instead of cardiac surgeons in a less invasive setting. Having the option of interventional over surgical procedures means a reduction in overall treatment costs as well as shorter recovery periods and hospital stays for patients. Some interventional cardiology procedures are described in the following sections.

Percutaneous Transluminal Coronary Angioplasty

Percutaneous transluminal coronary angioplasty (PTCA) has become the treatment of choice for many advanced cases of coronary artery disease. This procedure is performed by inserting an inflatable, fluid-filled balloon catheter into a coronary artery that is obstructed (usually not completely) by atherosclerotic plaque. After positioning the balloon catheter across the obstructive lesion (using fluoroscopy), the physician inflates the balloon, causing the plaque material to dilate or tear and compress closer to and into the walls of the coronary artery. This causes the artery to widen so that the blood supply to the heart is replenished.

This procedure may require initially using a balloon of narrow diameter to enlarge the narrowed vessel lumen, followed by a balloon larger in diameter. This variation allows the physician to enlarge the vessel lumen incrementally so as to minimize the risk of vessel rupture and achieve optimal opening.

Thrombolytic Therapy

During the past several years, physicians have had at their disposal thrombolytic pharmaceutical products. These drugs are used to dissolve blood clots, known as thrombi, that have *recently* formed in a patient's vasculature. The specific use discussed here is related to treating clot development in the coronary arteries. Because the clot must be treated shortly after it forms, thrombolytic agents are administered on an emergency basis.

Until the FDA's release of tissue plasminogen activator (t-PA) as a drug, streptokinase had been the thrombolytic drug of choice; urokinase, another early thrombolytic agent, was used less frequently. When emergency evaluation determines that the onset of chest pain, the patient's clinical status, and contraindications correlate to a carefully prepared protocol, the patient receives appropriate dosages of t-PA. Studies are under way that, once completed, could make it possible for qualified paramedics to administer thrombolytic drugs in the field. Like other recent technologies (such as MRI), t-PA is expensive; to date, Medicare has taken an extremely conservative posture on reimbursements for its use.

The release of findings from an extensive study on thrombolytic drug therapy has questioned conventional attitudes regarding the effectiveness of t-PA versus streptokinase. The study showed that overall these drugs have very similar success statistics (*Journal of the American College of Cardiology,* March 1991). However, there is tremendous cost difference between them—t-PA costs nearly 10 times as much as streptokinase. Despite the reported findings, debate continues regarding the clinical effectiveness and cost-effectiveness of one drug over the other.

Pacemaker Implantation

Several cardiac conduction abnormalities can now be treated by implanting permanent pacemaker devices. Historically, pacemakers were used to treat conditions related to abnormally slow heart rates. Today implantable systems treat certain rapid heart rate conditions and counteract other abnormal rhythm occurrences. Many of these very sophisticated devices are implanted routinely in patients in cardiac catheterization laboratories. The procedure requires fluoroscopic imaging of the pacemaker leads as they are being placed, and cardiac catheterization laboratories generally have high-quality fluoroscopic systems that are tuned to chest- and heart-imaging criteria.

In addition, implanting procedures have been refined so that they require only minor surgery to create the subcutaneous "pocket" for pacemaker generator placement. Placement of the pacing lead (or leads) can be accomplished by entering a large vein adjacent to the generator pocket using a needle and guiding wire system. Once located and functioning correctly, these lead wires are sutured securely at the point of vein entry, the generator is fully connected and checked, and the pocket is sutured closed.

Catheter Ablation

Catheter ablation is an essentially therapeutic electrophysiology (EP) procedure. Upon having diagnosed an abnormal cardiac conduction system and having located a malfunctioning vascular bundle, an electrophysiologist can treat some cases with catheter-induced ablation.

Ablation involves positioning an electrode catheter at the site of the abnormal conduction bundle and delivering up to 200 joules of electrical energy to the site through the catheter. The high current will cause the surrounding tissue to scar and the abnormal bundle to lose its ability to conduct the cardiac signal. This procedure is generally performed with a cardiac surgery team standing by in case of complications.

Valvuloplasty

The recent development of balloon valvuloplasty has led to several invasive cardiology programs offering this procedure in lieu of certain surgical procedures on selected patients. Developed in France, valvuloplasty involves the insertion of a large fluid-filled balloon catheter system to enlarge the orifice of stenotic (constricted) cardiac valves. A similar version of this procedure has been used to open congenitally restricted pulmonic valves and restriction associated with coarctation (narrowing) of the aorta.

After evaluating the patient's cardiac valve by echocardiography and standard cardiac catheterization, a physician chooses valvuloplasty only when specific criteria are satisfied. A primary criterion is whether the patient's cardiac valve is significantly calcified; valvular calcification can embolize as a result of the procedure and create arterial obstructions "downstream" from the valve, which may cause strokes or blockage of a peripheral artery.

A successful valvuloplasty can save the patient from undergoing open-heart surgery, which generally is performed for these types of conditions.

Both cost and length of stay are reduced dramatically with these procedures versus cardiac surgery.

Pericardial Centesis

Pericardial centesis is rare in most hospitals. The procedure involves inserting a large-gauge needle into the pericardial sac that surrounds the heart to drain excess fluid. This fluid accumulation may occur as a result of chest injury or, more often, as a symptom of certain forms of cancer or related side effects of cancer treatment. The catheterization laboratory fluoroscopic imaging system provides superior imaging capability during the needle insertion and fluid drainage.

Cardiac Surgery Interventions

The first cardiac surgical techniques developed corrected congenital cardiac defects. As diagnostic technologies improved for identifying adult heart disease, so too did surgical techniques. This section describes some of the more common cardiac surgery procedures performed under contemporary cardiac surgery programs.

Coronary Artery Bypass Graft

Coronary artery bypass graft (CABG) is the most frequent cardiac procedure performed in this country. Approximately 353,000 surgeries were performed in 1988.[1] This is nearly one-tenth of 1 percent of the nation's population in one year.

During CABG surgery, the purpose of which is to improve blood supply to the heart, the surgeon removes a segment of superficial vein from the patient's leg(s) and grafts the vein from the ascending aorta to a point past the obstructive lesion in a coronary artery. The "grafted" vein becomes a new conduit to supply arterial blood directly from the patient's aorta, past the obstruction, and to the heart muscle. This technique also can be used for multiple obstructed vessels. In one variation, the patient's internal mammary artery, rather than a vein graft, is used as the source of blood. This allows for the use of arterial tissue, which, unlike venous tissue, has been shown to be less susceptible to rapid reobstruction from atherosclerosis. This procedure requires the use of the heart–lung bypass pump (extracorporeal cardiopulmonary support).

Valve Replacement and Repair

Cardiac valve replacement has been performed successfully and effectively for several years. It requires the surgeon to remove a malfunctioning cardiac valve and to correctly fit and implant (sew into place) an artificial one. Artificial cardiac valves are either mechanical or biological. Mechanical valves are designed and constructed from nontissue components. Biological (bioprosthetic) valves are constructed of a combination of biologic tissue and nontissue components. Common biologic tissue components are derived from chemically processed bovine (cow) or porcine (pig) cardiac valve tissue.

Cardiac valve repair surgery is commonly categorized into two types of procedures: stenotic valve repair and insufficient cardiac valve repair. Valvular commissurotomies are procedures that relieve cardiac valvular stenosis. Surgical repair for insufficient valve (that is, the valve leaks when closed) requires the surgeon to "take a tuck" in the valve tissue and the valve ring (annulus), which amounts to tightening the valve to correct for insufficient blood flow. As is common for all open-heart procedures, the patient is placed on cardiopulmonary bypass during cardiac valve surgery.

Automatic Implantable Cardioverter/Defibrillator

The automatic implantable cardioverter/defibrillator (AICD) is a device that constantly monitors the patient's cardiac rhythm to detect potentially fatal cardiac arrhythmias, ventricular fibrillation, or ventricular tachycardia. If an irregularity is detected, the AICD delivers a burst of electric energy to convert the abnormal cardiac rhythm to a normal rhythm. This implantation procedure is used in patients with severe cardiac arrhythmias that cannot be controlled by drug therapy.

Cardiac Transplantation

Once performed only in select research hospitals internationally, cardiac transplantation is emerging in a number of large, urban cardiac surgery facilities. Even so, it is still a rarity compared with other cardiac surgical procedures. This is due to a number of obstacles:

- Unavailability of suitable organ donors
- Unavailability or shortage of mechanisms needed to surgically "harvest" donor hearts (or hearts and lungs)
- Inefficient means of transporting the organ(s) safely and in a timely fashion
- Incompatibility between transplanted organ(s) and recipient

Artificial Implantation

The past several years have seen the development of artificial implantable cardiac devices—specifically hearts and pumping devices called left ventricular assist devices (LVADs), which help the biological heart pump blood.

Rarely is a complete artificial heart implanted surgically. In most cases, heart implantation is an interim measure that provides a terminally ill cardiac patient with a life-sustaining device while he or she is waiting for a suitable donor organ. This technology has received tremendous media exposure and remains controversial.

Left ventricular assist devices are more common. The most familiar LVAD is the intra-aortic balloon pump (IABP), used in most coronary care units and postcardiac surgery units. This device consists of a large, fluid-filled balloon attached to a catheter, which is inserted into the patient's femoral artery and guided to a position within the descending aorta. The catheter is connected to the pumping system, which, upon receiving information from the patient's ECG, rapidly inflates and deflates the balloon "in sync" with the patient's heart contraction to pump blood *and* reduce the pressure that the left ventricle must generate.

Left ventricular assist devices are used to reduce the amount of injury a patient's heart may experience due to a myocardial infarction. They also are used to assist a heart severely impaired from other circumstances (for example, cardiogenic shock due to severe valvular dysfunction or infection).

Recent LVADs are actually surgically implantable pump systems with external power sources such as the IABP. This type of LVAD requires the surgeon to surgically insert the pump unit into the patient's aorta, where the device provides a pumping boost for the patient's own heart. Still under research development, these devices appear promising for those patients severely debilitated from reduced cardiac output.

Congenital Heart Disease Interventions

Repair surgery for congenital cardiac defects was among the first procedures developed. Today, several interventions are routine worldwide in pediatric cardiac surgery centers to treat the following conditions: atrial septal defect (ASD), ventricular septal defect (VSD), coarctation of the aorta, patent ductus arteriosus (PDA), tetralogy of Fallot, and transposition of the great vessels. Many of these conditions require complex surgical interventions, some of which are being performed on tiny infant hearts. Correspondingly, the mortality and morbidity statistics for this category of cardiac surgery are significantly higher than for adult cardiac surgery.

Historically, many congenital surgeries involved rerouting the patient's blood supply through the surgical insertion of patches, baffles, and conduits. Today, many of these procedures are performed with the patient on cardiopulmonary bypass and involve correcting the abnormalities in a closer-to-normal fashion. Furthermore, because of the complexity and time intensity of the repair work, many patients are placed in deep hypothermia. This dramatic reduction of body temperature reduces the tissue's need for oxygen and provides the surgeon with the time required to perform the procedure. The use of deep hypothermia also requires the addition of neurologic monitoring (electroencephalography [EEG]) to guard against neurologic damage from the reduction of body temperature.

Recent Developments and Ongoing Research

Several promising technologies that may have significant impact on both diagnostic and therapeutic cardiology are in various stages of research and development. Typically, these modalities are nearly all based on complex and expensive technologies that are equipment and education intensive. The following sections describe several of these new modalities and their potential role in diagnosing or treating cardiac disease. Their competitive and operational implications for cardiology departments also are discussed.

Laser Angioplasty

The development of laser angioplasty systems for the removal of coronary artery obstructions has been similar to that of balloon angioplasty (PTCA) procedures and products. Initial research and product development has been in the peripheral vascular field, with progress and technique evolving through work with the larger peripheral arteries. Currently, two major avenues of technology are being explored and developed: *thermal laser* and *excimer laser* systems.

The classical approach to laser applications is to use energy produced by the laser for its thermal (heat) component. The first attempts to apply laser energy for occlusive vascular disease correction used the heat energy approach by directing laser energy through a fiberoptic bundle to atherosclerotic plaque. Observers found that the area treated received extensive thermal damage and the fiberoptic tip frequently became coated with burned tissue. By adding a metal cap (known as a "hot tip") to the fiberoptic bundle, researchers created a heated cauterizing point that could be advanced through certain atherosclerotic lesions by searing through the tissue. This modification allowed more control of the heat source, thus causing less thermal tissue damage and minimizing damage caused by tissue collection on the tip.

Another laser device uses the laser energy to heat a metal tip that has a small, lens-covered port, which allows approximately 15 percent of the energy to pass through and directly irradiate the lesion. Also under development is a system that uses a hot tip but derives its heat from radiofrequency energy heating a gold tip. Similar experimental results have been obtained using the gold tip as with the more expensive laser hot tip systems.

The hot tip systems are on the decline in coronary artery applications. Although these systems enjoyed moderate success for peripheral arterial procedures, the complications they engender have caused researchers to look to other emerging technologies.

Another direction of laser angioplasty research and development is in the use of excimer lasers, sometimes known as "cool lasers." With excimer laser technology, tissue disruptions not caused by the same thermal energy delivery process to the tissue. Although their efficacy has not been fully proven, it is thought that the pulsed energy nature of excimer lasers may cause tissue destruction by breaking down the molecular bonds within the tissue. An alternative theory is that thermal energy is key but in an extremely localized region that does not show heat damage patterns similar to those of thermal laser and hot tip laser systems.

Over the past few years excimer laser systems have been approved for experimental use on human coronary arteries and have been used on peripheral arterial lesions with a high degree of success, although with somewhat limited experience to date. The promise of this technology is that it may eventually offer a safer and potentially more successful approach to the treatment of coronary artery disease.

Atherectomy Devices

In recent years, considerable research has focused on mechanical devices to remove coronary artery obstructions. This category of technology, given the name "atherectomy" due to its ability to remove plaque obstructions, is a contrast to the widening and compressive methodology used by conventional balloon angioplasty.

These devices vary significantly in design — from tissue-shaving systems, with an attached collection capsule for the removed tissue, to a very high-speed rotary blade unit, which virtually emulsifies the obstructive lesion into tiny pieces so as not to cause "downstream" blockages.

Ongoing research with these devices has shown them to be somewhat effective and, when used appropriately, to have an effectiveness and complication rate similar to conventional balloon angioplasty. Atherectomy is an emerging technology that continues to show promise and may become a significant interventional technique in the future.

Staged Thrombolytic Therapy/PTCA

For a number of patients, thrombolytic therapy for acute myocardial infarction (AMI) has proved to be highly effective for the reduction or reversal of the infarction process (see earlier discussion under "Therapeutic or Interventional Invasive Procedures"). In addition to treating AMI patients with thrombolytic drugs, physicians at several centers have followed this procedure with PTCA if the thrombolytic drug did not alleviate AMI. Staged thrombolytic therapy involves an emergency cardiac catheterization procedure shortly after admission for AMI. For a patient whose AMI episode ended with successful thrombolytic treatment, the elective scheduling of a diagnostic cardiac catheterization one to two days postadmission allows the cardiologist to evaluate the patient's coronary artery anatomy. Depending on its results, this diagnostic study may result in an electively scheduled PTCA or CABG procedure.

This combination of pharmaceutical regimens and invasive cardiology procedures has been recognized as effective for many patients in minimizing the possibility of a repeat acute myocardial infarction after successful thrombolysis. The procedure requires cardiac surgical standby capacity, because the potential for complications may be increased for recent AMI patients.

Coronary Artery Stents

Coronary artery stent insertion as a therapeutic procedure has been under investigation for several years. A stent is a device that is inserted into the patient's artery through a delivery catheter to prevent blockage of the vessel at that point. Various designs of vascular stents have included a coiled spring-like device and a cylindrical mesh unit.

Originally developed for peripheral and renal vascular applications, stents have been used in some investigating centers as "bailout" devices for failed PTCA procedures. Successful stent insertion at the point of a coronary artery dissection caused by PTCA may save the patient from emergency CABG surgery and could result in the long-term delay of surgery.

Ongoing research is under way to study the combination of PTCA and elective stent insertion at the point of angioplasty balloon dilatation to prevent or reduce re-stenosis of the patient's coronary artery. Current results are somewhat favorable and point to this technology as a potential interventional cardiology procedure.

Ultrafast

Ultrafast or Cine C/T™ is a computerized tomographic scanning technology that incorporates a steerable electron beam to produce X rays rather than the conventional, mechanically rotated X-ray tube and detector systems. By magnetically "steering" this electron beam to produce X rays, the system can acquire tomographic images very rapidly. Current systems can completely image one "slice" of the patient's body and change to the next imaging position in approximately 33 msec (a millisecond is one-thousandth of a second). This speed is similar to the 30 frames per second of cineradiography; hence the use of the Cine C/T™ name. This imaging speed is fast enough to "freeze-frame" the cardiac motion in a manner similar to cardiac catheterization.

With an imaging acquisition time of 33 msec, the Cine C/T™ unit can generate more than 30 "sliced" images of a patient's heart per second. These images are stored in a computer, which assists in analysis of the information recorded. Once a complete series of cardiac images is recorded, the computerized capabilities of the system allow the physician and technologist to create a three-dimensional stack of the individual "slices"; calculate cardiac chamber volumes at rest and during contraction; image and evaluate all intracardiac structures; and, with the use of contrast material injected into the patient's peripheral vein, possibly measure the blood flow through the coronary arteries and heart muscle tissue.

One advantage of this rapid scanning CT system is its ability to image moving body parts at such a high rate that motion artifact is reduced significantly or eliminated. In addition to imaging of the heart and other moving parts of the body, these units can produce the full spectrum of regular CT images.

Applications of Cardiac Magnetic Resonance Imaging

Until recently, the promise shown by magnetic resonance imaging (MRI) was not realized effectively because of inherent technical difficulties with MRI in acquiring images of moving anatomical parts. These problems were due to slow acquisition time (5–7 seconds) and the patient's heart rate (complete cardiac cycle 1–2 times per second), which would cause significant motion distortion.

Over the past two years, considerable progress has been made in reducing acquisition time, so that MRI has begun to show itself as a valuable and accurate tool for cardiac imaging. New computer-assisted capabilities allow for complete image acquisition within 40 msec. Fast magnetic resonance scanning has enabled the recording of three-dimensional cardiac images, the assessment of cardiac wall motion, and the determination of cardiac valve insufficiency—and to do so at procedural charge rates comparable to nuclear cardiac studies. Users of cine MRI technology now predict that eventually it could replace nuclear imaging for testing ventricular function at rest.

Freestanding Cardiac Catheterization Centers

Freestanding cardiac catheterization centers can be one of two kinds: laboratories located in hospitals that themselves offer no cardiac surgery services or laboratories located in a discrete facility that is neither attached to, nor operated by, a hospital. Cardiac catheterization laboratories in hospitals without surgery backup are now fairly common; "true" freestanding centers are less common.

So-called freestanding catheterization facilities are disallowed in many states. In others, however, not only are they approved but diagnostic cardiac procedures also can be performed in radiologists' offices. Some states are studying the advisability of these centers under pilot projects sponsored by state legislatures. In California, for example, a pilot project calls for the development of seven freestanding catheterization laboratories throughout the state. The laboratories may not be owned outright by hospitals, nor may they be operated on hospital-licensed property. The intent of this controversial legislation is to test the safety and efficiency of this alternative delivery system in a controlled environment. The project is overseen by the California Office of Statewide Health Planning and Development, which monitors program quality through a physician-staffed technical advisory committee. Stringent standards have been developed by this committee for the review of cases and granting of privileges to cardiologists who perform procedures in pilot facilities.

A freestanding center is an appropriate consideration for a hospital under two general strategic circumstances: as an effort to penetrate a new market area or as a joint venture to bond physicians to the hospital's catheterization program. Because non–hospital-affiliated freestanding centers may appeal to physicians, defensive promotion may be in order.

In this country, successful freestanding catheterization laboratories are built around one cardiologist or one cardiology group. Although there are some exceptions, for the most part this plan results in the smoothest operational environment — certainly the most profitable in terms of volume. The break-even point (in number of patients) can be lower for freestanding facilities because they open their doors under less stringent regulations in terms of building and operations.

Historically, Medicare did not reimburse facility fees associated with freestanding, non–hospital-affiliated catheterization laboratories. However, this situation has changed recently.

The future of freestanding catheterization laboratories will follow catheterization in general in terms of the impact of interventional catheterization and the need for standby cardiac surgical services. If in most states the cardiac surgery standard of practice remains intact and if there is parallel growth in therapeutic services and diagnostic procedures, then cardiologists will be less drawn to a freestanding center — despite attractions such as financial return or improved convenience for physicians or patients. There may be a growth in the postsurgical, vein graft patency evaluation market, however, that could be well served by these centers.

Mobile Cardiac Catheterization Laboratories

Mobile cardiac catheterization laboratories have been developed primarily for use during the refurbishing of existing laboratories or during the construction of new facilities. The technology is essentially the same as that available for mobile CT and mobile MRI services. Oftentimes, rural areas can afford access to cardiac catheterization only through these "labs on wheels," where the equipment is installed in a tractor–trailer rig and moved from location to location.

The technical and professional staff may be provided by the local hospital or by the service. Staffing needs for a mobile lab are determined by the local volume, regional requirements, and purpose of the facility. For example, a rural setting for which the mobile technology is a new service generally will import the technical staff. If a hospital's catheterization laboratory is undergoing renovation or if the hospital is adding a new service (invasive cardiology, for example) and is using a mobile unit until the permanent facility is constructed, generally that hospital will supply its own staff.

A pilot project similar to the one for freestanding catheterization facilities has been initiated by the California legislature to study the appropriateness and efficacy of this delivery system.

Some states either do not allow or otherwise regulate mobile catheterization. The competitive, technical, and safety concerns are similar to those noted for freestanding laboratories except where the mobile service is an interim arrangement at an established facility with an existing cardiac surgery program. Rural areas, however, may be well served with this technology, and rural hospitals should consider joint venturing with other hospitals or cardiologists as an alternative strategy in their development of cardiology services.

Although many mobile catheterization programs may succeed, others surely will fail. Failure will be tied to specific factors:

- Resistance to the concept among members of the medical community
- Failure of the hospital's medical staff to follow up on postcatheterization patients who use mobile laboratories
- Conflicts over scheduling
- Resentment toward the mobile cardiologist
- Insufficient demand or disagreements regarding levels of participation
- Inequitable distribution of program revenues

Successful mobile units either avoid or resolve these issues.

Summary

Diagnostic and therapeutic cardiovascular procedures are technology based and continue to trend toward less-invasive procedures. They depend initially on noninvasive technologies (EKG or TEE), which increasingly are available on an outpatient basis. Consequently, many hospitals find themselves in direct competition with local cardiologists or even with their own medical directors.

Noninvasive diagnostic technologies include echocardiology, stress EKG, ambulatory EKG (Holter monitoring), and a number of modes of cardiac ultrasound, called echocardiography/cardiac Doppler.

Invasive diagnostic procedures include cardiac catheterization and electrophysiology, which is also used therapeutically. Other less-invasive procedures under investigation are high-speed CT and MRI.

Therapeutic or interventional technologies include PTCA, pacemaker implantation, catheter ablation, thrombolytic therapy, valvuloplasty, and pericardial centesis.

Cardiac surgery interventions include CABG, valve replacement/repair, AICD, cardiac transplantation (heart transplant), artificial device implantation (LVAD, including IABP), interventions for congenital heart defects (such as ASD, USD, PDA, and tetralogy of Fallot).

Some technologies still undergoing research have potential for diagnostic and therapeutic applications. These include laser angioplasty, atherectomy devices, thrombolytic therapy combined with PTCA (against myocardial infarction), coronary artery stents, ultrafast or Cine C/T™, and cine MRI.

Freestanding catheterization centers can be located in hospitals that have no cardiac surgery services or in separate facilities that have no hospital affiliation. Mobile catheterization laboratories serve as interim facilities for existing labs under renovation or for new facilities under construction. They also serve some rural areas that otherwise would have no access to cardiac catheterization. Some mobile catheterization units are prohibited under state law unless they are affiliated with an established facility.

As the treatment of cardiac disease continues to shift toward interventional cardiology techniques as opposed to conventional cardiac surgery methods, utilization and status of cardiac surgery methods and of the cardiac catheterization laboratory continue to grow. At the same time, many current and emerging technologies are in competition with the catheterization laboratory for the diagnosis of cardiac disease.

□ Reference

1. *Heart and Stroke Facts.* Dallas, TX: American Heart Association, 1991, p. 17.

Chapter 10

Cardiovascular Services Facilities and Equipment

Finding the appropriate match between technology and facilities to provide optimal cardiovascular services is essential to a successful program. Whether a facility is expanding a noninvasive program or adding a new surgery service, certain unique issues related to facilities development must be addressed. This chapter identifies those issues—space design and allocation, equipment and furnishings, adjacency to other hospital services, and so forth. This way planners can position a program successfully, given its distinctive constraints, opportunities, and options.

Development of a Space Design Program

Planning any new or expanded clinical service should start with a comprehensive market assessment, as described earlier in this book. Market assessment results should yield projections for what program volume can be anticipated. These data allow for appropriate sizing of new or expanded facilities.

Armed with patient admissions and volume-by-procedure projections, the planner or planning group next develops a *space design program* tailored to these services. Space design, an important and often misunderstood component of facilities development, is meant to identify what physical areas are required to deliver the anticipated service(s) and how much space will be required. Physical space requirements are based on these factors:

- Program volume projections
- Basic program parameters (what services or procedures will be provided)

- Service space adjacencies (what nearby support services are needed as defined by clinical requirements)
- Regional building requirements
- Special user requirements

Once finalized, the space design program becomes the "blueprint," an inventory of all spaces needed for a project.

Optimal space design and allocation are achieved when appropriate clinical, management, and administrative staff work cooperatively with the architectural team. The architectural staff brings its expertise and knowledge of general facilities development and code requirements to the process, and the hospital staff identifies the clinical and operational needs of the planned program.

Ideally, the space for a new service should be developed within guidelines established through a hospital facilities *master plan*. The master plan is the result of a comprehensive study, usually undertaken with an architectural firm, that catalogs and details all the hospital's facilities development projects over the near and long term. The master planning process also should include a strong strategic planning component, which will assist the hospital planner (or planning group) in defining future physical plant development and how new services will be integrated into the physical plant. In the absence of a master plan, the design should be developed so as to anticipate—to the extent possible—future projects and minimize conflicts over space.

Table 10-1 is a sample space design program for a new, dedicated cardiac catheterization laboratory, a new cardiac surgery operating suite, and a cardiovascular surgery intensive care unit (CSICU). Note that this program only catalogs the required physical spaces, anticipated area (square footage) for each service, and necessary adjacencies or functional amenities. Once it is approved by the appropriate physicians, medical staff, and administrative constituencies, the completed program becomes the guiding document for design of the new services.

The design process for new or renovated facilities should begin with the *schematic phase,* which translates documented space needs (defined by the space design program) into conceptual *zones* or *blocks*. The schematic drawing includes all the rooms necessary to the project; however, because this stage is intended to work out adjacency and flow concepts, it does not provide details—actual room dimensions, doorways, and so forth. The schematic design stage allows the architectural staff to allocate "block" spaces for each service as defined by the design program. Detail is then translated to this block format.

Ideally, the schematic drawing is developed collaboratively with architectural staff and hospital staff so that general layout issues or conflicts can be resolved before proceeding to the time-consuming (and costly) final design

Table 10-1. Sample Cardiovascular Services Space Design Program

Facility	Square Feet	Comments
Cardiac Catheterization Laboratory		
Procedure room	550	
Control room	200	
Workroom/film review area	200	Shared between cath labs
MD's dressing area		
Scrub sink area	15	Could be in alcove of corridor
Equipment room	200	Shared between cath labs
Pre/postprocedure holding	150	
Cine film-processing room	125	
Staff dressing area/toilet	120	
Storage	150	
Manager's office/secretary	90	
Utility area	100	
Cardiovascular Surgery Operating Room		
Operating room	650	
Pump room (perfusion service workroom)	100	
Workroom	100	
Storeroom	100	
Scrub sink area	30	Three sinks minimum
Janitor's closets	50	Shared with CSICU and cath labs
Dressing facilities	250	Per male/female dressing facility
Staff toilets	40	
Supervisor's station	80	
Sterile supply	100	
Storage area	100	
Stretcher storage space	40	
Cardiovascular Surgery Intensive Care Unit		
Four critical care patient rooms	225 per room	Includes one isolation area with handwashing facility and utility area
Centralized nursing station	40	Includes space for desk, charting, lockable meds cabinet, refrigerator, handwashing fixture
Clean utility room	60	
Soiled utility room	60	
Janitor's closet	50	Shared with cath lab and cardiovascular surgery
Medication and storage preparation area	60	
Consultation room	75	
Public toilet	50	
Staff locker/lounge area	150	
Supplies storage area	120	
General Support Spaces		
Conference room	180	
Waiting room	100	Shared with other departments

stage. Frequently the schematic phase may generate several proposed layouts and reviews as conceptual issues are identified and fine-tuned. These repeat reviews should include the architectural team and the end user (hospital staff), the ultimate goal being to define general layout for each room and corridor within the plan.

Following review and completion of the schematic phase, the next step should be the *final design/development stage*. This process finalizes each room, corridor, and other associated spaces into complete architectural plans. These plans include detailed elevation and ceiling layouts for all areas.

Facilities Requirements

Facilities planning for cardiovascular programs revolves around the three major treatment/diagnostic areas: the cardiac catheterization laboratory, the cardiovascular surgery department, and the cardiovascular intensive care unit. Although these units may be planned separately and involve different staff, they must be considered within the framework of the hospital's master plan and the short-term and long-term projections for the entire cardiovascular program.

Cardiac Catheterization Laboratory

The dedicated invasive cardiology department or cardiac catheterization laboratory requires several support spaces that should be considered in planning space. The *procedure room* must be large enough to accommodate the radiographic system as well as provide work space and a supply/storage room for the physicians and staff. It also should be large enough to accommodate future upgrades of equipment; a common error in planning and developing a catheterization laboratory is failure to factor in space for future upgrades. For example, it is common to purchase a single-plane radiographic system for a new lab. Adding the second imaging plane (biplane conversion) often requires that an extensive structural steel system be installed in the procedure room ceiling. If at original installation the hospital also contracts for future upgrades and incorporates these contingencies in the structural, electrical, and mechanical systems, the upgrading time and expense will be minimized. Future space and systems technologies that can be anticipated in the planning include biplane radiographic capability, a digital imaging upgrade, and vascular laser systems.

When there is more than one procedure room, each should have a dedicated *control room* that is adjacent to the procedure room. The control room should house the main radiographic system controls and the main physiologic monitoring system. Locating these systems in a shielded control room, with clear visibility via a leaded window, removes staff members from the primary radiation environment and minimizes procedure room traffic during cases. This design requires installation of a dedicated intercom system for the control room and procedure room to ensure good communication between these areas.

Also adjoining the (main) procedure room should be a *clean setup room.* This room allows staff to prepare the sterile supplies for the next procedure in a clean environment, either prior to the completion of the previous case or during the turnover period between procedures. The clean setup room should be designed to include high-capacity, efficient supply/storage cabinetry.

The clean setup room, combined with the *preprocedure and postprocedure patient holding room,* will allow a single procedure room to accommodate annual volume of 900 to 1,000 cases before experiencing schedule overload. The patient holding room also serves as a preprocedure and postprocedure patient care area. The holding area should provide two holding beds for each procedure room. After the catheterization procedure is completed, the patient may be taken to this area to have catheters or sheaths withdrawn and a sterile dressing applied. Meanwhile, other staff members could be preparing the procedure room for the next case.

In addition to these specific space allocations, other support spaces may be necessary or recommended. For example, a dedicated catheterization laboratory requires a film-processing darkroom, a workroom/film review area for physicians, a film and procedural record storage area, staff dressing rooms with toilets, and a utility area to process soiled instruments and equipment postprocedurally. Other support areas may include a staff break/lounge area (which may be shared with another nearby department), a supervisor's office, an additional storage room adjoining the procedure room, and an equipment room to house the radiographic system components. Figure 10-1 shows a sample schematic (block format) design of a recently developed cardiac catheterization laboratory.

Cardiovascular Surgery Department

The major determinant of the cardiovascular surgery facility design will be whether the service will be a component of the hospital's main surgery department or will stand alone as a discrete, dedicated department. Many hospitals are developing dedicated cardiovascular operating rooms as a part of a complete cardiovascular services unit scheme. However, if the existing surgery department can accommodate the expansion required by a cardiovascular surgery service and if requisite service adjacencies can be preserved, staffing and operational economies of scale can be achieved by linkage to the hospital's main surgery department.

The cardiovascular surgery *operating room,* whether developed within the surgery department or as a dedicated cardiac unit, needs certain support

Figure 10-1. Schematic Design for Cardiac Catheterization Laboratory

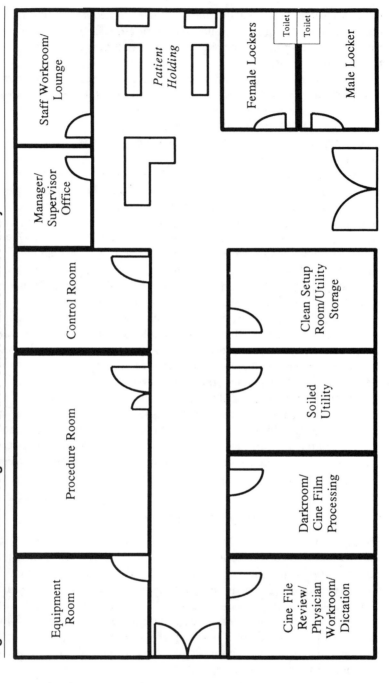

areas. A perfusion service workroom should be included close to or adjoining the operating room. This area, frequently identified as the "pump room," provides space for preparing the perfusion pump (heart–lung machine), storing perfusion supplies, and serving as the perfusionist's office/workroom.

Cardiovascular surgery requires extensive equipment and supplies, which necessitate a dedicated storeroom adjacent, or as close as possible, to the cardiovascular operating room. Each operating room should have an adjacent scrub sink area with consideration given to installing a three-way scrub sink.

A dedicated, stand-alone surgery service will require the addition of a number of support spaces, which in many cases will duplicate the main surgery department. These areas include storage for clean and soiled linen; sterile supply/storage; staff dressing facilities, including toilets; janitor's closets; a workroom for communications and paperwork processing; and an instrument storage area, which should include a rapid sterilizer. In addition, a staff break room/lounge and a department supervisor's office may be needed. Figure 10-2 depicts a sample schematic layout for a dedicated cardiovascular surgery department.

Cardiovascular Intensive Care Unit

The evolution of postcardiac surgery recovery facilities has mandated that this stage of care be provided in a cardiovascular surgical intensive care unit (CSICU). Many facilities have developed dedicated postcardiac surgical care units, whereas others have accommodated this service through using existing critical care beds and upgrading the physiologic monitoring system for beds in the unit. These combined critical care units may also care for other cardiac patients, general ICU patients, or other critical postoperative patients (neurosurgery, trauma, and so forth).

The CSICU is essentially a dedicated surgical intensive care department. As such, much of the required support spaces and design will reflect contemporary nursing service expectations for room size, adjacency, and storage in this area.

The critical care patient rooms must be large enough to accommodate the patient bed, the ventilator, and all other emergency equipment required for critical care. This equipment includes an intra-aortic balloon pump (IABP), left ventricular assist device (LVAD), cardiopulmonary support (CPS) system, and so forth.

An additional consideration for patient room size is that cardiovascular patients routinely have diagnostic tests performed, ranging from chest X rays to echocardiography and nuclear imaging studies. A nuclear scintillation camera is a massive unit requiring several square feet of floor space.

Additional support spaces for the CSICU include the centralized nursing station with space for paperwork processing and central station physiologic

Figure 10-2. Schematic Layout for a Dedicated Cardiovascular Surgery Department

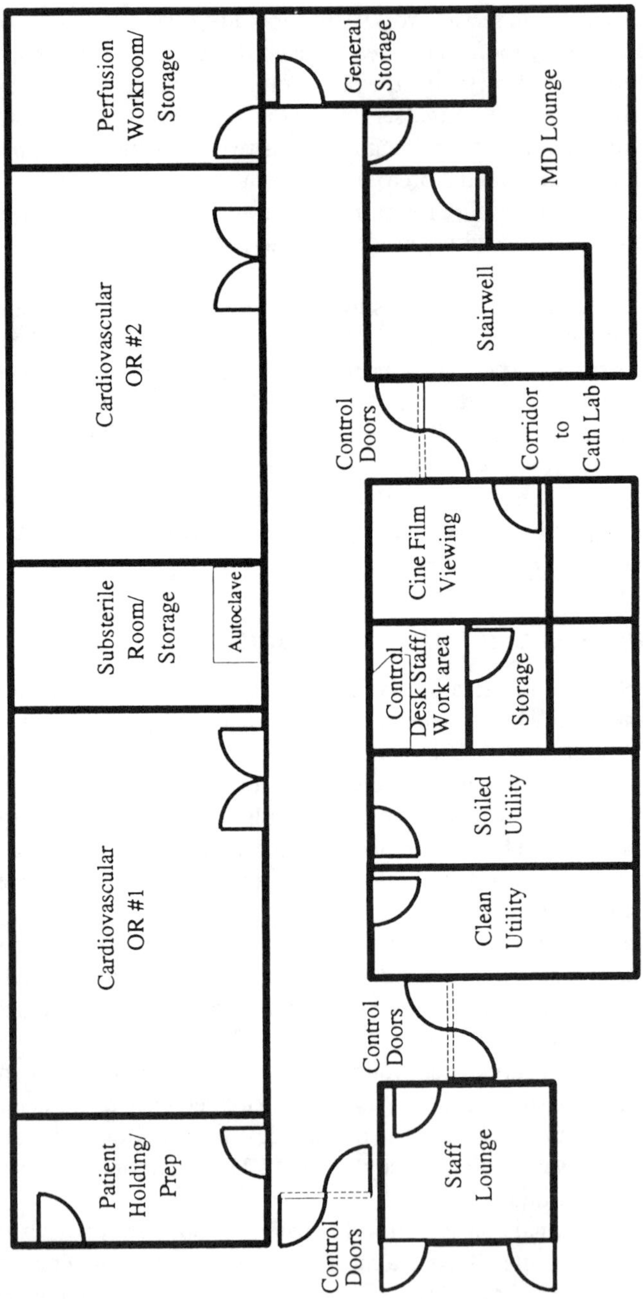

monitoring and charting; utility rooms for clean and soiled linen; a medication storage and preparation area; and staff locker/lounge area (for a stand-alone unit).

Nursing care units require a family waiting room, which ideally would be near the CSICU but may need to be located elsewhere in the hospital depending on space availability. A waiting room on another floor could work if there were good communications between the nursing unit and the waiting room via telephone or intercom.

Figure 10-3 is an example of a recently developed CSICU from a hospital that, due to space constraints, chose to establish a compact, four-bed intensive care unit. During construction, the 268-bed facility built in an extra shelled-in floor for future expansion.

Adjacency Requirements and Recommendations

Many clinical services must be developed in close proximity to each other, a condition referred to as an *adjacency requirement*. Adjacency requirements must be identified during the initial phases of facility development, particularly the space programming and schematic phases, to ensure appropriate placement of services.

Because occasionally it is necessary to transport interventional cardiology patients directly from the catheterization laboratory to the cardiac surgery department, the laboratory should be positioned as close as possible to the cardiac surgery suite to avoid transporting patients over long distances.

A new program must also minimize the distance between the CSICU for postoperative surgery patients and the cardiovascular operating room (CVOR). Postoperative patients often are unstable and may be connected to intravenous infusion lines, physiologic monitoring lines, and life-support systems. Therefore, patient transfer from the CVOR to the CSICU can be a formidable operation in itself. Add in the personnel and equipment necessary to effect this transfer — easily three or four staff members, the patient in a full-size bed with four infusion pumps, an IABP unit, and the anesthesiologist ventilating the patient for respiratory support — and the need for adjacency between the CSICU and CVOR becomes apparent. If these two areas cannot be contiguous, then plans should keep corridor travel distance to less than 200 to 300 feet.

In addition to postoperative patient transfer, the hospital must plan for emergency patient transfer back to the CVOR from the CSICU. Emergency situations generally are due to postoperative bleeding complications. The time and distance involved in returning a patient to the CVOR in an emergency usually are significant factors in the cardiovascular surgeon's evaluation of the program's facility development plan.

Figure 10-3. Schematic Design for a Dedicated CSICU

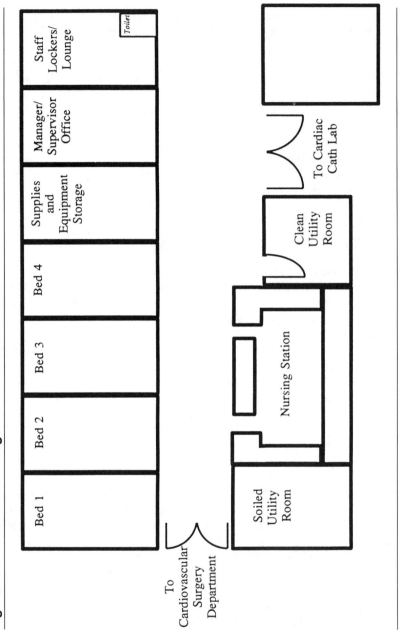

Historically, the CVOR was developed as a part of the hospital's main surgery department, but many newer programs have established their dedicated CVORs as separate, stand-alone departments. This recent trend is due to several problems associated with keeping cardiac surgery part of the main surgery department:

- The department lacks scheduling capacity.
- The department has no rooms large enough to house the required surgical technology.
- The department cannot accommodate adjacency between the cardiac catheterization laboratory and the surgery suite or between the CSICU unit and the CVOR.

These circumstances have also led many hospitals to develop a complete cardiovascular services unit, which houses the dedicated catheterization laboratory(ies), the surgery operating room(s), the surgery intensive care unit, and required support spaces for each of these services.

Whenever a hospital is forced to establish these new services in separate areas, even on separate floors, patient transport requirements must be accounted for. The staff and equipment requirements for postoperative patient transfer from the CVOR to the CSICU call for a large elevator cab. Patient transfer between floors can be ruled out in some circumstances due to unacceptable elevator conditions. Conversely, a large elevator that operates smoothly and provides direct floor-to-floor service can compensate for the CVOR and CSICU being several floors apart *if necessary.*

Ideally, the operating room and catheterization laboratory would be situated on the same floor adjoining each other. If insurmountable conditions make this plan impracticable, the best option is to minimize transfer distance and time and to avoid traversing public corridors.

Program Equipment Requirements

Providing cardiovascular services requires an extensive assortment of specialized high-technology equipment. Equipment ranges from high-resolution radiographic systems to complex perfusion systems (heart–lung units) that sustain life during cardiac surgery. Tables 10-2 (p. 240), 10-3 (p. 242), and 10-4 (p. 243) represent generic lists of equipment requirements for primary care cardiac-related departments, assuming a full-service program. The lists also show representative quantities, location assignments, and equipment prices (current as of this writing).

Two excellent sources for locating vendors for specific equipment are the *Health Devices Source Book,* published by ECRI, Plymouth Meeting, Pennsylvania, and the *Operating Room Product Directory,* published by the Association of Operating Room Nurses, Denver.

Table 10-2. Cardiovascular Surgery Department Equipment List

Room Description	Associated Equipment	Quantity	Price
Cardiac surgery	OR table w/attachments	1	$22,500.00
OR	Ceiling-mounted OR lights	1	$67,680.00
	Physiologic monitoring system	1	$58,000.00
	Slave monitor; color, 19"	2	$12,400.00
	Ceiling mounts for slave monitors	2	$4,800.00
	Gas/power columns	2	$14,000.00
	Recessed IV tracks	1	$2,500.00
	Sternal saw	1	$22,440.00
	Vascular instrument set	1	$25,000.00
	Heart/chest instrument set	1	$25,000.00
	Valve instrument set	1	$25,000.00
	Bring back instrument set	1	$10,000.00
	Electrosurgical cautery unit	1	$8,000.00
	Monitor/Defibrillator	1	$8,225.00
	SS table, 34" × 60"	1	$852.00
	SS table, 20" × 36"	1	$326.00
	SS table, 24" × 48"	1	$465.00
	Georgetown table	1	$850.00
	George table	1	$650.00
	IV poles	4	$784.00
	Kick bucket	2	$316.00
	Mayo stand	2	$704.00
	Sitting stool	4	$832.00
	Single basin stand	2	$464.00
	Fiberoptic headlight	1	$8,800.00
	Light source	1	$7,600.00
	Perfusion system	1	$80,000.00
	In-line blood gas monitoring system	1	$25,335.00
	Cell saver	1	$23,500.00
	Left ventricular assist device	1	$35,500.00
	Temporary pacemaker, single chamber	1	$4,000.00
	Temporary pacemaker, AV sequential	1	$6,000.00
	Fully equipped crash cart	1	$1,500.00
	Viewbox	2	$660.00
	X-ray and chart holder	1	$124.00
	Wastebaskets	2	$268.00
	Med storage cabinet	1	$500.00
	Intra-aortic balloon pump	1	$37,500.00
	Anesthesia machine	1	$70,000.00
	Anesthesia meds cart	1	$400.00
	NIBP for anesthesia	1	$2,500.00
	Infusion pumps	4	$12,000.00
	Transport monitor	1	$4,500.00
	Sitting stool	1	$208.00
	Solution warmer, dual compartment	1	$3,831.00
	SS table accessory cabinet	1	$2,517.00
	SS w/glass doors supply cabinet	2	$5,342.00
	SS desk unit w/drawers, sloping writing surface, bulletin board, and light	1	$2,872.00

Table 10-2. (Continued)

Room Description	Associated Equipment	Quantity	Price
Cardiac surgery OR *(continued)*	Stereo system with speakers	1	$1,000.00
	Wall clock	1	$50.00
	Time/elapsed time clock	1	$1,100.00
	Battery-operated emergency light pack	1	$170.00
	Heparin/protamine dosage system	1	$23,500.00
	ACT unit	1	$2,600.00
Substerile corridor	Scrub sink; SS, three-basin, knee-activated water and soap dispenser	1	$6,500.00
	Warming cabinet	1	$5,061.00
	Cine film projector	1	$16,900.00
	Steam sterilizer	1	$38,152.00
	Viewbox	2	$330.00
Perfusion storage	Storage carts	1	$1,000.00
	Blood bank refrigerator	1	$3,200.00
	Pharmaceutical refrigerator	1	$4,500.00
	Total cardiac surgery equipment		$751,308.00

Summary

Planning facilities (plant and equipment) for a new or expanded cardiovascular program begins with developing a space design program based on a market assessment. The program should include input from key clinical, management, and hospital administrative staff. The design process begins with the schematic phase, which translates the space needs into facility blocks or zones; this phase helps planners work out adjacency and other work flow issues prior to beginning more costly work. The next phase finalizes the design, and specific architectural details are filled in.

Facilities for a full cardiovascular program include a catheterization laboratory, a surgery department, and an intensive care unit. Although requirements for these facilities vary, both short-term and long-term program goals, as well as adjacency issues, should be considered carefully. Ideally, all of the areas will be on one floor and pose no transfer barriers from one to the other.

Equipment requirements vary for specific cardiovascular programs. Equipment inventory, price, and location assignment should be assessed cooperatively among relevant staff users.

As with other planning processes described in this book, cardiovascular facilities planning requires the input of clinical and medical staff.

Table 10-3. Cardiac Catheterization Laboratory Equipment List

Room Description	Associated Equipment	Quantity	Price
Viewing area	Cine film projector	1	$16,900.00
	Cine film storage cabinet	1	$1,000.00
Darkroom	Cine film processor	1	$22,200.00
	Densitometer/Sensitometer	1	$3,500.00
	Film splicer	1	$339.00
	Film processor automixer	2	$3,600.00
	Cardiovascular phantom kit	1	$1,162.00
Alcove/utility	Scrub sink—2-basin; knee-activated water and soap dispenser	1	$6,500.00
	Blanket warming cabinet	1	$5,061.00
	Apron holders	2	$380.00
Control room	Leaded glass window; 6' × 3'	1	$4,500.00
	Physiologic monitoring system	1	$150,000.00
	Sitting stool	2	$416.00
	Intercom system to cath lab	1	$3,000.00
Cath lab/special procedures	Radiographic system with digital imaging	1	$1,100,000.00
	Oximeter	1	$9,300.00
	Intra-aortic balloon pump	2	$37,500.00
	Contrast injector	1	$19,900.00
	Vascular Doppler	1	$800.00
	Instrument tables, 34" × 60"	3	$1,500.00
	Monitor/defibrillator w/external pacing	1	$10,000.00
	Crash cart with all instruments, meds, etc.	1	$1,500.00
	Temporary pacemaker	1	$1,000.00
	Cardiac output computer	1	$1,200.00
	Digital elapsed time clock	1	$1,100.00
	Lead aprons	8	$1,500.00
	Lead thyroid collars	2	$120.00
	Leaded glasses	2	$340.00
	Controlled medication lockbox	1	$250.00
	Stereo equipment	1	$1,000.00
	Battery-powered emergency light unit	1	$119.00
	Total cardiac cath lab equipment		$1,405,687.00

Table 10-4. Cardiovascular Surgery Intensive Care Unit

Room Number	Associated Equipment	Quantity	Price
Room 1	ICU bed	1	$1580–3800
	Overbed table	1	$386
	Bedside cabinet	1	$550
	Patient chair, high-back	1	$800
	Patient chair, regular	1	$350
	Bedside physiologic monitoring unit	1	$26,000
	Sphygmomanometer, wall-mounted	1	$105
	Otoscope/opthalmoscope, wall-mounted	1	$600
	Headwall system with medical gases, electrical outlets, and suction	1	$1000–2500
	Bedside commode	1	$5800
	Procedure lighting	1	$103
	Cubicle curtain track and curtain	1	$100
	IV track, ceiling mounted	1	$100
Room 2	ICU bed	1	$1580–3800
	Overbed table	1	$386
	Bedside cabinet	1	$550
	Patient chair, high-back	1	$800
	Patient chair, regular	1	$350
	Bedside physiologic monitoring unit	1	$26,000
	Sphygmomanometer, wall-mounted	1	$105
	Otoscope/opthalmoscope, wall-mounted	1	$600
	Headwall system with medical gases, electrical outlets and suction	1	$1000–2500
	Bedside commode	1	$5800
	Procedure lighting	1	$103
	Cubicle curtain track and curtain	1	$100
	IV track, ceiling mounted	1	$100
Room 3	ICU bed	1	$1580–3800
	Overbed table	1	$386
	Bedside cabinet	1	$550
	Patient chair, high-back	1	$800
	Patient chair, regular	1	$350
	Bedside physiologic monitoring unit	1	$26,000
	Sphygmomanometer, wall-mounted	1	$105
	Otoscope/opthalmoscope, wall-mounted	1	$600
	Headwall system with medical gases, electrical outlets, and suction	1	$1000–2500
	Bedside commode	1	$5800
	Procedure lighting	1	$103
	Cubicle curtain track and curtain	1	$100
	IV track, ceiling-mounted	1	$100
Room 4	ICU bed	1	$1580–3800
	Overbed table	1	$386
	Bedside cabinet	1	$550

(Continued on next page)

Table 10-4. (Continued)

Room Number	Associated Equipment	Quantity	Price
Room 4	Patient chair, high-back	1	$800
(continued)	Patient chair, regular	1	$350
	Bedside physiologic monitoring unit	1	$26,000
	Sphygmomanometer, wall-mounted	1	$105
	Otoscope/opthalmoscope, wall-mounted	1	$600
	Headwall system with medical gases,		
	electrical outlets, and suction	1	$1000–2500
	Bedside commode	1	$5800
	Procedure lighting	1	$103
	Cubicle curtain track and curtain	1	$100
	IV track, ceiling mounted	1	$100
Nursing station	Central station for physiologic monitoring		
	system	1	$32,000
	Remodel NS casework		
CCU general	Intra-aortic balloon pump	1	$37,718
equipment	Infusion pumps	16	$2100–3400
	Mobile IV poles	4	$209
	Total CSICU equipment		$221,923–250,523

Chapter 11

Case Studies

The six case studies that follow highlight various aspects of the planning and management of cardiovascular services. It is important to note that (1) no one planning, development, or implementation strategy works in every situation, (2) every program is different, and (3) the opportunities and problems are unique to individual facilities. Therefore, the challenge for planners and managers is to match strategies with specific environments and solutions with specific circumstances.

Although every situation is unique, some principles in the management of specialty services can be applied in a general way to most situations. These principles are discussed in each of the cases.

Case 1 (General Medical Center) identifies steps in the development of a clinical pathing method and standard treatment protocols for a cardiovascular program in a large tertiary care facility. Case 2 (Crestview Memorial Hospital and Northside Hospital) illustrates how the competitive relationships between two hospitals changed when an inpatient surgeon moved from one hospital's cardiovascular program to the other's. Case 3 (New West Memorial Hospital) describes how a large community hospital maintained its market position in cardiovascular services by establishing a heart institute through a joint venture agreement with two dominant cardiology groups. Case 4 (Browning Medical Center and Whitney Hospital) illustrates how a hospital that consistently was second in market share in a two-hospital town established itself as dominant in the cardiology market by first developing a cardiac catheterization laboratory. Case 5 (Hazelton Hospital) indicates what happens when the community and the hospital's medical staff create a political barrier to a new cardiac program, in this case cardiac surgery. Case 6 (Mountain Hospital) describes how a failing cardiovascular program was given new direction by a group of cardiologists who shared a common vision.

Case 1: General Medical Center

General Medical Center (GMC) is a 400-bed tertiary care facility specializing in cardiovascular, neuromuscular, and other specialty services. The hospital serves an urban and semirural market area (100-mile radius) in the Midwest.

In 1989 cardiovascular services utilization volume was 675 cardiovascular surgeries, 4,500 cardiac catheterizations, and 1,200 percutaneous transluminal coronary angioplasties.

The hospital has been considered high priced, with a total average case charge for CV surgery of $37,000, one of the highest in the state. To control costs and per case charges, GMC used a clinical pathing methodology on five key cardiovascular DRGs (104, 105, 106, 107, and 112) to create standard treatment protocols (STPs) that would enhance the efficiency and effectiveness of clinical care while decreasing both costs and charges per case. *Clinical paths* are the combination of patient care practices that are the most resource efficient and clinically appropriate for a particular medical condition or procedure and that result in the shortest length of stay. The following provides an overview of the process and the outcome of the clinical pathing and protocol development efforts at GMC.

Feasibility Analysis

A two-part analytical process was conducted to determine the value and feasibility of developing a standard treatment protocol and whether standards could help decrease charges and enhance market position with managed care contractors.

The external market assessment included surveying employers, insurers, consultants, insurance brokers, and employer coalitions, as well as interviewing hospital managers and physicians. This process resulted in preliminary data on the level of demand, desired pricing, potential opportunities, possible competitors, market barriers, and so forth.

An internal analysis ascertained the expected level of administrative and physician participation in the clinical pathing process. The analysis also reviewed the following: financial position and operating budgets and possible financial impact of clinical pathing; strategic planning documents; and utilization statistics, current charges, and costing methodologies. It was concluded that potential existed for decreasing the average charge for CV surgery cases.

A computer-based financial model was developed to create line-item-specific charge and cost information for each of the DRGs targeted. A "typical" patient profile was based on a detailed audit of a sample of representative patient hospital bills for each target DRG. This model allowed for detailed analysis of charges and a basic understanding of resource consumption to be used for purposes of clinical pathing and standardization.

General Medical Center wanted to identify which changes in standard patient treatment (for example, decreasing the number of EKGs per case from the current average of four to an average of three) would result in significant savings per case when totaled for each patient. The hospital had no cost-accounting system in place at the time; therefore, the cost analysis was limited.

The feasibility analysis concluded that the opportunity identified in the market assessment justified developing the STPs and continuing on to full development. One conclusion reached was that the target rate per DRG to be utilized in the internal development process should be approximately a 30 percent discount off current charges so as to be competitive with other providers of similar services.

Protocol Development

A small group of physicians—cardiovascular surgeons, cardiologists, and anesthesiologists—were designated to participate in the development of the standard treatment protocols and in the eventual development of contractual relationships with payers. The task of developing STPs for cardiovascular surgery was assigned to a task force of nine multidisciplinary committees. These committees consisted of representatives from all departments affected and included the steering committee of hospital administration, the cardiovascular protocol committee (CPC), and seven subcommittees in specialized areas including surgery, critical care, nursing units, cardiology, pharmacy, central supply, and laboratory. The goals were as follows:

- Review and document the clinical path for each target DRG and match current cost and charge information.
- Review existing protocols and standing orders.
- Establish a standard patient selection and screening process.
- Produce a new protocol and standing orders, comparing and contrasting new costs and charge implications with target rates.
- Quantify annual savings and calculate cost and charge per case, and compare with target rates.
- Determine ongoing protocol revision, monitoring process, and schedule.
- Produce an implementation plan for the protocol.

The hospital assigned a member of administration to serve as project coordinator. The coordinator, assisted by two staff members of the consultation team, divided staff support among the committees.

Documenting the clinical path of a typical patient through the system, from preadmission testing to discharge, was integral to the protocol development process. The concept of clinical pathing implies three other conditions:

1. *Clinical appropriateness:* Only those tests and procedures are performed that are clearly dictated by the patient's condition or specified in an STP.
2. *Efficiency:* The patient is provided the necessary services when, during his or her clinical course of treatment, those services will produce the greatest medical benefit by the medical personnel most suited to providing the most cost-effective care.
3. *Quality:* Quality is measured both in terms of demonstrable clinical outcome (for example, comparative mortality and morbidity rates) and a high level of patient satisfaction.

Each subcommittee prepared a clinical path for patients utilizing their nursing unit or specialty area. A target average length of stay for each DRG was calculated by the CPC and substituted for the historical length of stay (for example, from 18 days for DRG 104, to a target of 10 days), and the clinical path was then analyzed and amended to conform to project goals and objectives.

The subcommittees functioned with a spirit of cooperation and purpose not seen before at GMC. Issues and ideas surfaced that had never been shared before because there had been no multidisciplinary forum for them and, therefore, no framework for analyzing and correcting problems or taking advantage of opportunities identified. Thus, the process itself had implications far beyond the confines of the original tasks: It improved communications between clinicians and administrators.

The subcommittees recommended these changes, which subsequently were implemented:

- *Preadmission testing:* Set up a method to schedule extensive preadmission testing and patient education before the day of admission so as to save one day of stay for a surgical patient.
- *Standing orders:* Revise uniform standing orders for pre- and postcatheterization and PTCA to result in more appropriate treatment, higher patient satisfaction, and decreased average costs and charges.
- *Diagnostic testing:* Decrease the average number of inpatient diagnostic tests (ECG, chest X ray) by setting a protocol for the number allowed.
- *Drugs:* Change pharmaceuticals commonly prescribed for surgical patients so as to eliminate inappropriate drugs, approve clinically acceptable and less expensive substitutes, and eliminate pharmaceutical practices considered wasteful or duplicative.
- *Patient satisfaction:* Establish a formalized exit interview procedure to ascertain levels of patient satisfaction with the program.
- *Laboratory tests:* Create a laboratory test panel that cuts out tests judged to be unnecessary.

- *Scheduling:* Change scheduling of PTCAs, CV surgery, and PTCA backup so as to increase efficiency and decrease waiting times.
- *Standardization:* Standardize products, tests, procedures, and so forth, to increase efficiency.
- *Appropriateness criteria:* Establish criteria to screen candidates for CV surgery and PTCA.
- *Physician quality standards:* Adopt physician quality standards (for example, measure the percentages of infection rate, postoperative bleeding, mortality, and PTCA success rate against a standard based on consensus.)
- *Patient furloughs:* Establish policies requiring patient furloughs in order to decrease the lengths of hospital stays — if a course of hospitalization can be interrupted.
- *Case prices:* Establish DRG-specific case prices, including hospital-specific and physician-specific components.
- *Role clarification:* Formalize clarification of physician roles regarding patient management so as to enhance efficiency and communication.
- *Costs:* Determine costs per procedure in lieu of a cost-accounting system, with the assistance of the hospital's finance department.
- *Patient education:* Prepare and videotape extensive pre- and post-surgical patient education programs.

Over a six-week period the subcommittees met every other week for two-hour meetings. Extensive informal meetings and research (for example, the appropriate use of Swan–Ganz catheters) took place as needed. The CPC met on alternate weeks to consider recommendations passed to it by the subcommittees, make changes to the recommendations, or send them back for reconsideration. In addition, the CPC became a clearinghouse for key issues that emerged as being critical to the project's success. Some of these included:

- Capacity of existing nursing units, particularly the monitored bed unit, to handle the projected increase in patient loads
- Physician issues related to whether to include physicians in the protocol development process and subsequent managed care contracting activities
- Mechanisms to ensure collaboration among surgeons and cardiologists to determine appropriate medical intervention (for example, surgery versus PTCA)
- Mechanisms for effective and timely patient transfer from nursing units

Consulting staff prepared a draft of the STPs (with supporting documentation and a clinical path for each target DRG), which they presented to the CPC for review. In addition, staff made various assumptions in the financial models for each DRG to determine, as accurately as possible, a typical patient bill, given the draft protocol. Although incomplete at this time, matching cost information also was presented.

The CPC expressed satisfaction with the process and the outcome to date and identified some areas that had "fallen through the cracks." Staff work continued to complete all documentation.

Protocol Implementation

Toward the end of the protocol development process, hospital and consulting staff prepared a protocol implementation plan. The draft was presented to the subcommittees and the CPC for review and comment.

Creation of the STP called for a detailed review of how patients are routinely treated at GMC. Implementation required not only the education of nurses and other personnel who must administer the protocol, but a patient identification system, changes in medical staff rules and regulations and in hospital policies, revised job descriptions and work assignments, and countless other procedures to ensure compliance. The plan also called for a series of forums to train personnel in protocol compliance and variance reporting, as well as the designation of a full-time protocol manager to supervise the protocol process.

The CPC created the protocol utilization committee (PUC), which was empowered to review all protocol patients for physician compliance, for medical or system-related variations in care, case charges, and overall patient satisfaction. Mortality and morbidity monitoring would continue through the mortality and morbidity conference. A standard data base on all protocol patients would be established and administrative reports issued to support the PUC's activities.

Results

The results of the activities at GMC have been impressive and have met original expectations. Following is a summary of significant results to date:

- *Costs, case charges, and case rates:* The protocol development process took approximately 60 days. Over this period, a 24 to 32 percent reduction in case rates and case charges for the targeted DRGs was achieved with a commensurate decrease in costs. Profit margins ranged from 20.5 percent to 36.1 percent. For example, in DRG 104, Cardiac Valve Procedure with Catheterization, the average case rate decreased 27.1 percent, from $42,977 to $31,330, with a profit margin of 27.1 percent. Table 11-1 compares average charges before and after STP. Over

Table 11-1. General Medical Center, Cardiovascular Surgery and PTCA: Initial Financial Results of STP Protocol

DRG	Pre-STP Average Charge	Post-STP Average Charge	Percentage Decrease	Total (Direct and Indirect) Cost	Percentage Margin	Medicare Rate
104	$42,977	$31,330	27.1	$23,434	25.2	$35,990
105	$35,723	$26,971	24.5	$20,709	23.2	$27,516
106	$34,689	$23,450	32.4	$18,624	20.6	$25,953
107	$27,490	$20,178	26.6	$16,042	20.5	$19,392
112 (PTCA)	$13,915	$10,631	23.6	$ 6,792	36.1	$ 8,767

Note: Figures include hospital costs and charges *only.*
Source: Used with permission of Ronning Management Group, Inc., 1990.

time, GMC intends to continue its cost-cutting activities in targeted areas and expects to decrease the costs per case even further.

* *Length of stay:* Length-of-stay standards were revised to 56 percent of the current average lengths of stay per DRG. For example, length of stay for DRG 104 decreased from an average of 18 days to 10 days; DRG 105, from 14 to 9 days; DRG 106, from 14 to 8 days; DRG 107, from 11 days to 7 days; and DRG 112 (PTCA), from 5.6 to 1.5 days. The decrease in length of stay resulted in a decrease in charges of over $5,500 per case for DRG 104, a total of 47.7 percent of the total decrease in charges per case.
* *Other charges:* Although decreases in average length of stay contributed 47.7 percent of the total decrease in DRG 104 charges per case, an additional $6,000, or 52.3 percent, of total charges per case was saved. For example, monitoring charges decreased 76.9 percent from an average of $2,808 per case to only $648 per case, and pharmacy charges decreased 42.0 percent from an average of $3,500 per case to $2,050 per case. Decreases in average charges were made in the vast majority of departments affected.

Conclusion

The process of clinical pathing implemented at GMC is ongoing and will continue to result in positive changes to the system. Progress continues to be made on refining elements of the system and further understanding the costs involved with all aspects of individual surgical cases. It is hoped that the STP and clinical path methodologies have given the hospital an effective instrument to continue to refine the cardiovascular surgery program and to find applications for other specialty programs as well.

Case 2: Crestview Memorial Hospital and Northside Hospital

Crestview Memorial Hospital (Crestview) and Northside Hospital (Northside), two urban hospitals in a large city in the West, have 405 and 390 beds, respectively. Located about a mile apart, they are tertiary hospitals offering comparable services to a wide geographic area. They have been extremely competitive; during the recent past, Northside consistently held a larger market share in most services.

Northside also has been the leading cardiovascular program provider in the area for many years, with volumes that position it not only as the statewide leader, but among the largest programs in its region. Crestview has respectable numbers for its cardiovascular program, but had attempted (unsuccessfully) for many years to build a dominant cardiovascular program.

Northside's cardiovascular program was established by a well-qualified and aggressive surgeon who has run the program since its inception more than 20 years ago. The surgical program developed a referral network of cardiologists and primary care physicians that extended for hundreds of miles. On the other hand, Crestview had relied principally on the referrals of cardiologists located in the immediate area.

The two hospitals competed aggressively in the managed care arena, with Northside occupying a clear leadership position because of its low-cost structure and the aggressive posture the surgeon had taken within the payer community as well as the multispecialty group community. Northside positioned itself as the "value leader," with low cost and high quality.

Crestview's Program Development

During the mid-1980s, Crestview Memorial Hospital underwent a change in management and began to focus on recruiting prominent cardiovascular physicians to the hospital staff. After establishing a strong team of new invasive and interventional cardiologists, Crestview successfully recruited Northside Hospital's principal surgeon.

Crestview achieved this coup not only because of its strong financial commitment to the surgeon, but because it was able to exploit the deteriorating relationship between the surgeon and Northside by emphasizing the growing cardiology department at Crestview. By offering the surgeon a physician-centered environment, Crestview was able to break up a 20-year relationship between the surgeon and Northside.

The results of the two hospitals' program development efforts are shown in table 11-2, which lists the cardiovascular procedure volume between 1984 and 1988. Three conclusions can be drawn from a review of these figures:

1. The cardiovascular surgery business at Crestview exploded between 1985 and 1987 and more than quadrupled by 1988, while the cardio-

Table 11-2. Results of Program Development Efforts

Facility/Procedure	1984	1985	1986	1987	1988
Crestview Memorial					
Catheterization	882	1,104	1,160	2,754	3,659
PTCA	5	91	116	426	681
CVS	278	290	434	1,081	1,226
Northside Hospital					
Catheterization	2,120	2,122	2,310	1,371	1,829
PTCA	187	240	293	313	284
CVS	1,341	1,282	1,167	786	778

vascular surgery volume at Northside fell by 40 percent between 1985 and 1988. This shift in volume is directly attributable to the cardiovascular surgeon's moving from Northside to Crestview.

2. The diagnostic cardiac catheterization volume, which was nearly three times as great at Northside in 1984, quadrupled between 1984 and 1988 at Crestview Memorial. This also is the direct result of Crestview's recruiting Northside's cardiovascular surgeon, as well as recruiting the strong team of invasive and interventional cardiologists.

3. Finally, although Crestview did not enter the PTCA market until 1984, by 1988 its cardiology team was doing more than double the PTCA volume being done by its competitor.

Conclusion

Northside Hospital maintains a respectable program volume, given the fact that one of its key surgeons defected from the cardiac surgery group.

These two hospitals, comparable in terms of location, facility, staffing, and administrative support services, have had remarkably different experiences in the cardiovascular market. In 1984, Northside was the clear and dominant leader, not only over Crestview but throughout the state. By 1988, Northside was no longer one of the top hospitals in the state, was dominated by Crestview Memorial Hospital locally, and had seen its once-valued position as the leader in cardiovascular services taken over by Crestview. These cataclysmic changes did not occur as the result of marketing, promotion, technology, facilities, staffing, or general management functions. This shift occurred entirely as the result of Crestview Memorial Hospital assembling the right team of physicians at the right time. Although not every hospital can imitate what Crestview did, the lesson to be learned is that high-quality specialty programs are created, and achieve volume when the franchise is built around the players.

Case 3: New West Memorial Hospital

New West Memorial Hospital (New West) is a 600-bed hospital located in
the Southwest in a community with a population of 2 million. The hospital
competes with the cardiovascular programs of two other facilities, one a
university hospital. New West historically has dominated cardiovascular services in this market, but administration sensed a need to consolidate its medical staff organization.

At the initiative of one of the cardiologists, the hospital, the two
dominant cardiology groups, and the surgery group forged a joint venture
agreement to develop a for-profit heart institute. The heart institute was developed to serve as a focal point to identify the cardiovascular program. It brings
the participants together for joint business planning and serves as the vehicle for a number of joint venture activities, including a diagnostic cardiology imaging center, a cardiac rehabilitation program, a health promotion
program, and a research program. The institute, which houses all of the
cardiovascular physicians' offices, is located on the hospital campus in a
separate building, which is owned by the joint venture.

The diagnostic services available at the heart institute represent a sharing of facilities by the cardiology groups that result in a substantially
improved profit margin for these services. However, these services duplicate
the noninvasive cardiology services available at the hospital.

The institute functions as the exclusive provider of professional services
for all cardiac patients at the hospital. This strategy was a result of evaluating the benefits gained from a mutually exclusive arrangement with these
physicians as opposed to negotiating with a numerous assortment of smaller
cardiology groups, independent cardiologists, and cardiovascular surgeons.
Even though a certain patient volume was given up, it was believed that in
the long run quality and costs could be managed better by a smaller group
of dedicated physicians and that an enhanced market share would materi-
alize. The Heart Institute at New West Memorial has become the clear market leader in cardiovascular services throughout the state.

The principal marketing focus of the group is management based on
physician-to-physician relationships. One physician functions as the principal source of contact between all referring physicians, a position that grew
out of this physician's natural networking abilities. Some direct consumer
marketing is done in order to establish and enhance consumer preference
for the institute.

New West's heart institute functions the way many cardiac institutes in
the future will operate. That is, it is based on exclusive relationships between
physicians and the hospital; it is located in a separate building owned by
the participants; and the participants are committed to building a program,
recognizing that individual practices will grow only as a result of the program's overall success.

Conclusion

New West has selected an exclusive physician distribution strategy that has been successful because of the size of the cardiology groups and their inherent competence. This approach will not work in every contemporary market, but it can be expected that the strategy will become the preferred model in the future. Cardiovascular services increasingly will compete on the basis of quality and cost. Because quality and case cost depend on physician practices, those programs that can team up with highly competent and resource-efficient physicians will gain market share in most markets. Creating an organization such as a heart institute to formalize relationships can be expected to become the norm.

Case 4: Browning Medical Center and Whitney Hospital

Browning Medical Center (BMC) historically held second place in market share for virtually all services in a two-hospital town drawing from a market area of about 250,000. Whitney Hospital, its competitor, was a more established facility that was owned by a religious order and was well funded and well run. Browning, on the other hand, was a former physician-owned hospital developed fairly recently and now owned by a proprietary chain. The medical community generally favored Whitney Hospital.

New Development

Several years ago Whitney Hospital denied the request of the town's sole cardiologist to establish a cardiac catheterization laboratory. Whitney Hospital felt that it was unnecessary and perhaps inappropriate to add catheterization services in this largely rural market, particularly with only one invasive cardiologist on staff.

Browning Medical Center seized the opportunity to develop a catheterization laboratory and did so quickly and aggressively. Soon the community found itself with three invasive cardiologists where there had been one, solely owing to making a catheterization laboratory available. Within 18 months, the catheterization laboratory patient volume had jumped from 500 to 1,100 patients annually.

Based on the volume in the new catheterization laboratory and the new cardiologists' leadership, discussions began at BMC regarding the viability of adding a cardiac surgery program. A surgery group from a nearby town, which had been the recipient of the referral volume from this community, expressed its eagerness to supply the surgical support necessary to initiate the program (rather than possibly lose patients to other surgeons). The cardiac surgery program was developed quickly, and the surgical volume soared along with an increasing volume of cardiac catheterization cases. At last count, BMC's annual catheterization laboratory volume was approaching 2,000 cases, the cardiac surgery volume was exceeding 500 cases, and the number of angioplasties exceeded 600 cases.

While BMC was seeing its cardiovascular business boom, it was also witnessing an extremely positive response to the cardiovascular program within the medical community and among the hospital staff. The success of the cardiovascular program contributed significantly to the higher spirits of the hospital staff, and morale soon soared to an all-time high.

The cardiovascular program also attracted some of the best nurses and technologists in town, who migrated from Whitney Hospital, which was witnessing sagging morale and decreasing volumes in its emergency room, its CCU, and across virtually every service line (see figure 11-1).

Conclusion

Where Browning Medical Center saw advances and increased volume, Whitney Hospital experienced declines. Because of an aggressive local marketing campaign by Browning, community attitudes changed regarding the two hospitals. Although Browning's efforts did not completely tip the scales in its favor, the two hospitals had become essentially equal competitors in the community where Whitney had once dominated. This appears to be a result of a combination of the cardiologists' unwillingness to provide services at Whitney because of its lack of sophisticated cardiovascular services and their awareness that their time is more efficiently spent at Browning Hospital. Consequently, the CCU at Whitney is not directed by a cardiologist, as is more common, but rather by an internist.

Because of the availability of cardiovascular services at Browning, local paramedics take all of their cases with suspected cardiovascular involvement to Browning. Because the cardiologists naturally favor Browning, a number of internists and general practitioners have begun admitting to Browning patients with cardiovascular or secondary cardiovascular conditions; they also have shifted their entire practices to Browning Hospital for reasons of convenience.

Being at the wrong end of the cardiac "value chain," Whitney Hospital had little choice but to add a cardiac catheterization laboratory and is in the process of adding cardiac surgery. It could be argued that the presence of two cardiovascular surgery programs in the town is unnecessary and duplicative, but a strong case also could be made that Whitney needed new development so that it could compete directly. Otherwise, it would have faced continual decline.

Figure 11-1. Whitney Hospital: Total Admissions to CSICU, 1983–1988

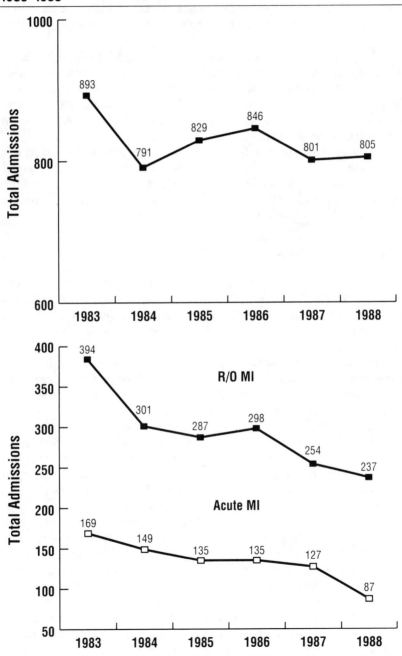

Case 5: Hazelton Hospital

All planned health care programs do not proceed to development. Insurmountable barriers can occur at any point in the planning stage, even during development.

Hazelton Hospital is a 215-bed hospital in the Midwest. It is located about an hour's drive from a major metropolitan area that has ample cardiovascular surgery services available from larger hospitals. Hazelton provides only basic cardiology services. The group of four cardiologists who serve Hazelton recently sponsored the installation of a cardiac catheterization laboratory in the hospital.

The same group pressed for development of cardiovascular surgery services on the basis that these services were not only appropriate to a regional referral center (such as Hazelton), but also necessary to the cardiologist desiring state-of-the-art facilities for interventional services. Hazelton, as the sole hospital facility in town, was willing to consider such a venture.

Feasibility Assessment

A feasibility assessment determined that cardiovascular surgery was *financially* viable. With an estimated volume approaching 200 surgeries during the initial year of operation, there appeared to be little financial risk. Volume was also expected to include nearly 200 angioplasties, which would add to the overall profitability of the program.

The feasibility assessment also included an evaluation of the hospital's physical facilities to clarify whether a new program could be implemented easily. The current facility was found to be constructed in such a way that cardiac surgery could be initiated with minimal capital additions or building expenditures.

The major barriers seemed to be the medical staff and the community. Hazelton is a "typical" community hospital with a medical staff that is well integrated into the community and that has traditional values. Although the medical staff is highly skilled, their attitudes regarding new program development are not particularly aggressive.

As the hospital considered the addition of cardiovascular surgery to its program offerings, a series of interviews was held with the medical staff and representatives of the community advisory board. The attitudes of the medical staff were mixed, with several physicians expressing strong reservations about the clinical viability of cardiovascular surgery at Hazelton Hospital. The community advisory board members expressed concern about potential duplication of services and the ability of the program to attract top-notch physicians. Subsequent to further discussions between the hospital planning committee and individual medical staff leaders, a determination was made to postpone the addition of cardiovascular surgery indefinitely.

Conclusion

The situation at Hazelton Hospital points out that although cardiovascular surgery programs can be economically feasible, operationally viable, and strategically supportable, without the political support of the community and medical staff, they will fail. The hospital staff neglected to consider the political forces within the community and medical staff and were unable to develop and implement a strategy to win support for the program.

Case 6: Mountain Hospital

Mountain Hospital is a 350-bed hospital located in a two-hospital semirural community on the West Coast. The local medical community is characterized by a large number of solo practitioners.

Program Evaluation

The hospital has had a cardiovascular program, including cardiovascular surgery, for a number of years. However, the program has languished with only moderate utilization compared to its crosstown rival.

After repeated analyses and investigations into the reasons for the program's lackluster performance, including extensive interviews with the medical staff, administration, and ancillary and support services staff, a number of themes, issues, and variables emerged. When the program was compared to a model program and to the flourishing crosstown rival, a number of deficiencies in structural variables and organizational elements were revealed.

After studying these factors, it was concluded that the program lacked the medical leadership and direction demonstrated in the model program and at the crosstown rival hospital. The cardiac surgeon was in solo practice, as were all of the cardiologists supporting this program. Within the program there was no forum, institute, or other organizational system for the regular processing of cardiac program business. The cardiac program suffered from a lack of identity, which in turn bred a lack of loyalty among and between the participants. All the cardiologists split patient admissions between both hospitals (although certain cardiologists admitted a majority to Mountain Hospital).

During the review process, three of the cardiologists stepped forward with an invitation to form a hospital-based cardiology group. As this process began to evolve, a surprising stabilization of political phenomena also took place. The cardiology program began to take on an identity of its own and was given direction by the new three-person group. A new unanimity formed among the cardiologists, the surgeon, and other support specialists.

Although initial program volumes did not skyrocket following this re-organization, there developed a sense of control, purpose, and destiny regarding the program and its potential success.

Conclusion

Clinical programs *must* be built around physicians dedicated to providing the leadership and direction necessary to give the program identity and the ability to function effectively.

Summary

These cases each make important points relevant to hospitals operating or developing cardiovascular programs:

- *Case 1:* Case costs can be managed successfully for competitive advantage through the use of a combination of a structured group process, modification of physician practice behaviors, identification of proper incentives, and the development of standard treatment protocols.
- *Case 2:* Successful programs are built around physicians the way that successful sports franchises are built around players. Marketing, facilities, and technology are important to the success of a program but no more so than the stadium and concessions are to a successful sports franchise.
- *Case 3:* Because the cardiovascular market is becoming increasingly competitive, quality and cost—both determined principally by physicians—are becoming more essential to program success. Therefore, successful programs secure exclusive arrangements with highly competent and resource-efficient physicians who will enhance their market position. The heart institute can be a powerful vehicle for promotion and, more important, for strengthening the bond between hospital and physicians.
- *Case 4:* Many communities lack cardiovascular programs or have only limited services. These services are being successfully developed at relatively low volumes, often generating more demand than projected. Not only can they be successful but the "cardiac food chain" can be devastating to competing hospitals that lose not only cardiac patients but other patients with cardiac disease as a comorbid condition.
- *Case 5:* Although some markets may be ready for the addition of cardiovascular surgery from financial, program, and strategic standpoints, neglecting political (community and medical staff) factors will doom the program. A strategy to address political issues must be incorporated early in the development process to ensure the program's long-term success.

- *Case 6:* Many cardiovascular programs have been, or are being, suffocated by cardiologist groups who endeavor to keep all competition out of the hospital, even at the expense of market share. There are also programs in which no group dominates. In both situations, the problem is lack of physician leadership and a lack of a program-centered vision. All programs benefit from strong physician leadership with a program perspective.

Chapter 12

Cardiovascular Institute Development

Cardiovascular institutes (also known as heart institutes) have become so popular an addition to hospitals that they constitute a nearly meaningless point of differentiation. Some communities find them attractive and others find them of questionable value, particularly when they do not deliver on what they imply—improved quality and research. Many institutes are nothing more than promotional vehicles that have little to show beyond a newsletter and a series of cocktail parties.

The principal value of cardiovascular institutes lies in their organizational structure. In the typical organization, the stakeholders within the program have no vehicle for addressing business concerns of the program or for bringing together physicians and managers who influence the organization. Neither the medical staff nor the administrative structure offers such opportunity.

A model for the traditional structure of a cardiovascular institute is shown in figure 12-1. In this model, the institute is owned by the same parent organization that owns the hospital and is organized around nonoperational activities such as fund-raising and education. Figure 12-2 illustrates a suggested model for an evolving institute. The key differences are the operational orientation and joint ownership of the institute. This joint ownership can involve either another hospital, one or more groups of physicians, or both. Although slow to develop, these arrangements have the potential to evolve into a modified "medical mall" concept. A third model involves an institute formed by a cardiovascular medical group to compete in many respects with its host hospital.

Whereas the operations components of the evolving model are yet to be determined, future conditions will call for these institutes to become increasingly operationally oriented, thereby forcing the participants into even

Figure 12-1. Cardiovascular Institute: Traditional Hospital Model

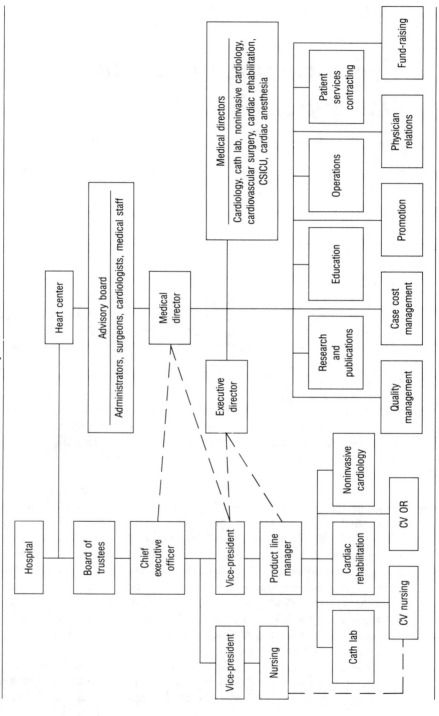

Figure 12-2. Model for an Evolving Cardiovascular Institute

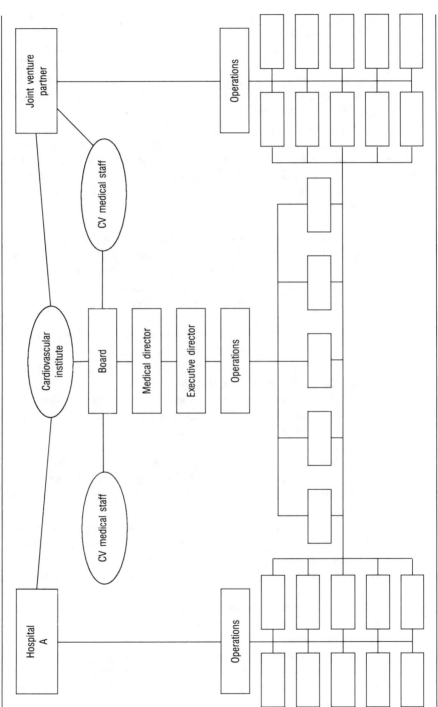

closer affiliation. This in turn will align members' goals and give rise to a truly "joint-ventured" program.

Developing an operationalized, joint-ventured cardiovascular institute cannot be done in one step. Table 12-1 presents a planning matrix that describes four scenarios across 12 structural variables. Three of the scenarios are assessed in table 12-2 (p. 268) against seven criteria. This assessment process helps determine the potential course of development for an institute. Appendix E is a business plan outline for development of a heart institute.

Figure 12-3 (p. 269) lists issues to be considered in preparing alternative scenarios. The medical staff, as well as the administrative staff and the governing board, should be involved in this process. After issues are evaluated, the results can be developed into a Concept Outline, which addresses (at a minimum) the following topics:

- *Mission:* The mission statement is a broad and general statement of purpose that sets the tone for discussion regarding the specifics of the institute. The questions that underlie any mission statement are *What purpose or objective will the organization serve?* and *What need will the organization meet in the market that is not presently being met?*
- *Role:* The role statement defines the position the institute will assume in the market, both externally and internally. The role statement attempts to operationalize the concepts in the mission statement.
- *Goals:* Goals identified for the institute should range from the general — statements regarding overall development of cardiovascular services and fund-raising — to the specific — forming strategic alliances among physician groups or between physician groups and the hospital.
- *Governing board:* The concept paper should discuss how the organization will be governed differently from the hospital or the program, specifically which institutions or groups will be represented and who will represent them.
- *Organizational structure:* The institute can take a variety of forms and can evolve from a simple fund-raising and promotional vehicle to a complex operation. The concept paper should address the initial organizational structure and, if not inflammatory, the potential for development.
- *Management:* Related to governance, the question of management concerns who will make things happen for, and throughout, the institute. This question should be addressed both from the administrative and the medical staff perspective. A variety of committees can be put in place to carry out the work of the institute early in its development; these committees can serve a purpose throughout the life of the institute.

Table 12-1. Heart Institute Development Options

Option	Scenario 1	Scenario 2	Scenario 3	Scenario 4
Identity	Separate heart institute identity/location	Separate heart institute identity/location	Separate identity/no separate heart institute location	No separate heart institute identity
Clinical research	Yes, self-funded	Yes, self-funded	Minimal	Minimal
Education/training	MD, RN, technician, public	MD, RN, technician, public	MD, RN, technician, public	Public
Fund-raising	Yes, institute directed	Yes, institute directed	Yes, hospital(s) directed	Yes, hospital(s) directed
STP/clinical path	Yes, quality + cost = value	Yes, quality + cost = value	Cost analysis	No (continued financial loss)
Packaging of services	• SPPO development • General contracting	• SPPO development • General contracting	• SPPO development • General contracting	Limited
Management/organization	See table 12-2			
Medical director/physician organization	See table 12-2			
Data system	Product line data system	Product line data system	Limited, nonspecific	Limited, nonspecific
Promotion	Based on substance • Payers • Primary care • MDs/cardiologists • Patients through PCMDs	Based on substance • Payers • Primary care • MDs/cardiologists • Patients through PDMDs	Market to payers, Medicare-eligible, primary care, MDs/cardiologists, patients through PCMDs	None
Primary care physician program	• Satisfaction • Communication • Affiliation/patient education	• Satisfaction • Communication • Affiliation/patient education	Affiliation/patient education	Affiliation/patient education
Cost	$100K—Institute CEO $75K—Product line manager $250K—Marketing and promotion (includes patient rep) $40K—Administrative assistant $35K—Data $60K—Consulting	$120K—STP $85K—Administration $150K—Director, marketing and promotion (includes patient rep) $35K—Administrative assistant $35K—Data	Percentage of salary $100K—Marketing and promotion (includes patient rep) $30K—Administrative assistant $15K—Administrative assistant $60K—Consulting	None

Table 12-2. Assumption Analysis

Criteria	Scenario 1	Scenario 2	Scenario 3
Value	Quality and price sells	Same	Same
Quality	Documentable	Same	Same
	Program is leader	Program is potentially superior	Program is competitive
Margin	HMO and Medicare can be profitable	Same	Increased volume will reduce loss
	Increased margin is available through STP/cost reduction	Same	Cost reduction via cost analysis
Market	HMO potentially jeopardizes other contracts available	Same	Same
	Opportunity to be leader	Same	
	Market void exists	Same	Same
Organization	Multisite	Focused	Part-time
Data	Information is powerful	Same	Same
Promotion	Requires substance	Same	Is necessary

- *Location:* Physical location is a key issue, particularly as it relates to the participation and support of specific physician groups. Special consideration should be given to the needs of the stakeholders.
- *Facilities:* Where the opportunities exist, physical facilities should be designated for the institute. Whereas such facilities initially relate primarily to administrative activities, opportunities often arise to create owned and operated facilities, such as a noninvasive and/or invasive cardiology diagnostic center or a cardiac rehabilitation program.
- *Staffing:* Access to staff should be provided early on (principally clerical staff) and, as the program becomes operational, technical and research staff can be added. Staffing and management needs may be revised as the concept paper progresses.
- *Finances:* The finances of the institute also will be clarified once its mission, role, and organizational structure begin to take shape. Although hospitals frequently fund the development of institutes, joint ventures can serve to bond physician groups to the project.
- *Target Markets:* As in any business development effort, it is important to understand the markets that will be served by the development efforts. In the case of a cardiovascular institute, an evaluation of the intended impact on the medical staff (including cardiologists, cardiovascular surgeons, and primary care referring physicians), the general public, business/industry, and third-party payers should be conducted. These target markets should be prioritized and the institute structured so as to maximize the impact on the high-priority markets.

Figure 12-3. Heart Institute Development (Scenario Issues)

1. Organization
   - Mission and role
   - Statement of operations (services provided directly, indirectly, relationship, etc.)
   - Legal structure (profit/nonprofit)
   - Advisory board composition, timing, and appointments (interim and permanent)
   - Committee/subcommittee composition, timing, and appointments

2. Medical Direction
   - Appointment of medical director
   - Duties of medical director
   - Reimbursement/salary to medical director

3. Physician Participation
   - Medical staff (inclusion versus exclusion)
   - Staff appointments
   - Committee/subcommittee structure, timing, and appointments

4. Administration
   - Integration of heart institute with operations
   - Administrative organization
   - Heart institute CEO/product line manager
   - Cardiology department manager
   - Integration of nursing units and personnel
   - Timing, recruitment, and appointments

5. Joint Venture Aspects
   - Joint-ventured catheterization laboratory
   - Joint venture concepts
   - Target venture partners
   - Sales plan, timetable, and implementation
   - Integration of joint venture heart institute into overall organization
   - Other joint venture opportunities

6. Programs and Services
   - Criteria for program development
   - Development of program/service opportunities
   - Selection of diversification activities, timetables, and implementation plans
   - Budgeting/funding of diversification opportunities

7. Physician Recruitment
   - Development of target list of physicians and physician groups
   - Development of recruitment plan
   - Allocation of resources (human and financial) for recruitment

8. Strategic Affiliations
   - Criteria for, and identification and evaluation of, affiliation opportunities
   - Hospital/heart institute affiliations
   - Physician joint ventures/affiliations
   - Payer/employer group affiliations

(Continued on next page)

Figure 12-3.   (Continued)

9. Cost/Quality/Volume Paradigm
    * Creation of standard treatment protocols for CV surgery
    * Establishment of quality standards and measures
    * Analysis of charges per case for CV surgery
    * Cost-reduction activities to reduce cost per case
    * Managed care contracting

10. Research
    * Research mission, goals, and objectives
    * Protocol for research proposal approval and funding
    * Funding of research

11. Education
    * Educational mission, goals, and objectives
    * Development of professional (physicians, nurses, technicians, etc.) educational component
    * Public education activities
    * Employer and payer education programs

12. Fund-Raising
    * Capital campaign for heart institute building and equipment
    * Fund-raising program for start-up and ongoing activities
    * Resource allocation (fund development, public relations, marketing, etc.)

13. Marketing
    * Integration of existing marketing activities
    * Allocation of resources (human and financial)

14. Annual Work Plan
    * Development
    * Budget development and adoption process
    * Utilization and role of outside consultants

15. Budget
    * Capital requirements
    * Operating budget
    * Fund-raising goals

---

* *Key Strategies:* An effort should be made to outline the key strategies to be used in the initial phases of the institute development process. The strategies will relate specifically to the form and structure the institute will take in the target markets identified. The more specific the strategies can be early in the process, the greater the potential for galvanizing interest and effort on the part of the participants.

These topics will lead to the creation of scenarios that vary the scope of each variable described above. As agreement is reached on the focus and direction of the institute, work can begin on preparation of the business plan. Although promotion will not be the only focus for the heart institute of the future, it will continue to be an important function. Table 12-3 includes an initial marketing and promotion budget that easily could be adapted for use by a cardiovascular program without an institute.

Summary

The development process for a cardiovascular institute as outlined in this chapter is not substantially different from the development process for other cardiovascular programs. The development of a cardiovascular institute requires a very close examination of the organization's goals and organizational structure as well as the role the institute will play in the market and other issues.

Table 12-3. Cardiovascular Institute: Projected Five-Year Operating Budget

Year	Hard Costs		Moderate Costs		Soft Costs		Totals
1	Initial set-up costs:		Marketing costs:		Radio talk program and ads	$2,220	
	Legal fees	$7,500	Publications	$21,200	Billboard	4,000	
	Logo	2,000	Direct mail campaign	27,000	Nursing seminar	2,000	
	Stationery	1,300	Advertising	35,465	Community education	5,000	
	Office space	5,100	Ad development	4,500	5K–10K plan	5,000	
	Equipment/furniture	9,000	MD seminar	5,220	Promotionals	19,395	
	Office supplies	2,500	Wellness clinic	12,000			
	Telephone	6,000	Mailing costs	$10,000			
	Salaries	132,500					
	Benefits	26,875					
		$192,775					
	Brochure development	30,000					
	Directory advertising	19,000					
	Bulk mail permit	250					
		$242,025		$115,385		$37,615	$395,025
2	Legal fees	$7,500	Marketing costs:		Direct mail (biannual including		
	Office space	5,100	Brochure reprint	$10,000	mailing costs to new residents)	$12,000	
	Office equipment	9,000	Publications	21,200	Talk program	2,220	
	Furniture/supplies	2,500	Wellness clinic	12,000	T-shirt replacement	6,000	
	Telephone	12,000	Advertising	34,965			
	Salaries/benefits	168,375	Community education	5,000			
	Bulk mail permit	50	MD seminar	5,220			
	Stationery	1,300	Mailing costs	10,000			
	Directory advertising	19,000					
		$224,825		$98,385		$20,220	$343,430

#			Marketing costs				Total
3	Same as year 2	$224,825	Publications	$21,200	Brochure request	$10,000	
	Development of new direct mail campaign	27,000	Wellness clinic	12,000	Talk program (biannual)	1,240	
			Advertising/new ad development	30,000	New promotional	3,000	
			MD seminar	5,220	T-shirt replacement	6,000	
			Community education	5,000			
			Mailing costs	10,000			
		$251,825		$83,420		$20,240	$355,485
4	Administrative costs	$224,825	Brochure reprint	$10,000	T-shirts	$6,000	
			Publications	16,200	Talk program	500	
			Wellness clinic/health fair	15,000			
			MD seminar	5,220			
			Advertising	20,000			
			Community education	2,500			
			Direct mail—new residents	10,000			
			Mailing costs	10,000			
		$224,825		$93,920		$6,500	$325,245
5	Administrative costs	$224,825	Publications	$21,200	5K–10K plan	$5,000	
			Wellness clinic	12,000	New promotional item	$3,000	
			MD seminar	5,220	Talk program	500	
			Advertising	20,000	Nursing seminar	2,000	
			Community education	2,500			
			Direct mail—new residents	10,000			
		$224,825		$80,920		$10,500	$316,245

Cardiovascular Surgery and Invasive Cardiology Services Business Plan

Table of Contents
 I. Executive Summary
    A. Summary of Recommendations, Program Objectives, and Program Description
    B. Market Analysis and Demand Projections
    C. Management and Organization
    D. Staffing Plan
    E. Medical Directorship and Medical Staff Issues
    F. Facilities and Equipment Requirements
    G. Financial Feasibility
 II. Program Description
    A. Services to Be Provided
    B. Service Benefits; Target Market
    C. Staffing of Service
    D. Overview of the Comprehensive Cardiovascular Services Program
 III. Market Analysis
    A. Market Area
    B. Population Trends and Demographics
    C. Utilization and Market Share Analysis
    D. Usage Rate Analysis
    E. Internal Trends Evaluation
    F. Summary and Conclusions
 IV. Program Start-up
    A. Capital Requirements
    B. Working Capital Requirements
    C. Program Start-up Staffing Requirements
    D. Legal Issues

E. Antitrust Issues
F. Regulatory and License Requirements
G. Required Contractual Arrangements
H. Medical Staff Issues
I. Project Time Frame
V. Marketing Strategy
A. Medical Staff and Community Attitudes
B. Positioning
C. Marketing Campaign and Promotional Activities
VI. Management and Organization
A. Cardiovascular Services Management
B. Administrative Responsibility for Cardiovascular Services
C. Implementation
VII. Operations
A. Facilities
B. Equipment
C. Service Capacity
D. Staffing Requirements
E. Staffing Level Projections
F. Departmental Productivity
G. Personnel Availability
H. Operational Expenses
I. Charity Care: Policies
J. Program Philosophy
VIII. Project Phasing
IX. Financial Projections
X. Program Evaluation

Cardiovascular Services Strategic Business Plan Outline

I. Executive Summary
   A. Description of Hospital and CV Project
   B. Site Location and Market(s) Area to Be Served
   C. Description of Cardiovascular Programs and Services
      1. Current program and services
      2. Proposed program and services
   D. Description of Facilities, Equipment, and Significant Technologies Involved
   E. Opportunities and Threats within the Market(s)
   F. CV Product Line Goals, Objectives, and Strategies
   G. Distinctive Characteristics of CV Program and Services
   H. Projected Sources and Uses of Funds
   I. Implementation Plan and Schedule
II. Market Analysis and Plan
   A. Description of Hospital/Product Line and Services
      1. Existing business/services
      2. Planned business/services
   B. General Description of the Industry
      1. Industry trends and assumptions
      2. Cardiovascular trends and assumptions
   C. Target Market Profiles and Description (Local/Regional, Primary/Secondary)
      1. Consumer market(s) identification, size, and trends
         a. Market, submarket identification
         b. Population and demographic analysis
         c. Profiles and trends
         d. Results of primary market research

      2. Physician market(s) identification, size, and trends
        a. Market, submarket identification
        b. Profiles and trends
        c. Results of primary market research
      3. Other market(s) identification, size, and trends (insurers, business/industry, etc.)
  D. Competitor Analysis (Existing/Potential)
      1. Hospital competitors
      2. Physician/medical group competitors
      3. Other competitors (as identified)
  E. Demand Forecasts/Projected Utilization
      1. Cardiology (diagnostic/therapeutic)
      2. Cardiovascular surgery
      3. Educational/community services
      4. Ancillary/supportive services
  F. Marketing Mix Analysis (Customer Motivation to Utilize)
      1. Product/service
        a. Consumer needs and service offering
        b. Quality issues
      2. Pricing
        a. Pricing strategies
        b. Packaging strategies
        c. Price versus cost
      3. Place/service delivery
        a. Location
        b. Marketing considerations of site(s) location
        c. Delivery mechanism (hours of operation, scheduling, physician referral system, etc.)
      4. Promotion/sales
        a. Promotional activities
        b. Sales plan (as required)
        c. Advertising and media selection
III. Human Resources Plan
  A. Management Team
  B. Management Staff Requirements
  C. Personnel Requirements
IV. Operations Analysis and Plan
  A. Geographic Location(s)
  B. Facilities
      1. Physical plant description
        a. Cardiovascular surgery
        b. Cardiology
        c. CSICU
        d. Ancillary/support services

        2. Technology assessment
        3. Capital equipment requirements
        4. Timetable and implementation
   C. Hours of Operation/Scheduling
   D. Patient/Physician Referral Systems
   E. Organization and Management
        1. Product line management
        2. Joint venture structure (as applicable)
   F. Timetable for Implementation
        1. New programs and services
           a. Cardiovascular surgery
           b. Cardiology
           c. Other
        2. Revised programs and services
   G. Critical Risks and Potential Problems
V. Financial Plan
   A. Business Financial Strategy
        1. Revenue enhancement
        2. Program and service development
        3. Technology procurement
        4. Physician recruitment and development
        5. Other
   B. Profit/Loss Statements for Three Years (with assumptions)
   C. Cash Flow for Three Years
   D. Budgets for Three Years (with assumptions)
   E. Capital Budgets
   F. Financial Reporting Mechanisms
   G. Other
VI. Appendixes

Appendix C

Cardiovascular Services Implementation Questionnaire

Department Name: _____ Department Number: _____

I. List any departmental comments and/or concerns you have regarding the addition of cardiovascular services and indicate any action required.

_____
_____
_____
_____
_____
_____
_____
_____
_____
_____

II. Personnel Requirements: The personnel section of this questionnaire corresponds directly to the incremental work hours that will be required to provide cardiovascular services.

A. Please write a brief explanation justifying the need for additional manhours required to implement and maintain adequate staffing levels.

_____
_____
_____
_____

B. Estimate number of total additional manhours required: _____
C. Types of positions (title) required:

	Description	Manhours (estimated)
1.	_____	_____
2.	_____	_____
3.	_____	_____
4.	_____	_____
5.	_____	_____
6.	_____	_____
7.	_____	_____
8.	_____	_____
9.	_____	_____
10.	_____	_____
11.	_____	_____
12.	_____	_____
13.	_____	_____
14.	_____	_____
15.	_____	_____
	Total	_____

III. Equipment Requirements: Identify any additional equipment needs in order to provide cardiovascular services:

	Description	Cost
1.	_____	_____
2.	_____	_____
3.	_____	_____
4.	_____	_____
5.	_____	_____
6.	_____	_____
7.	_____	_____
8.	_____	_____
9.	_____	_____
10.	_____	_____
11.	_____	_____
12.	_____	_____
13.	_____	_____
14.	_____	_____
15.	_____	_____

IV. Training/Education Requirements
   A. Are there any education requirements for your department that will need to be addressed prior to the opening of the cardiac center?   Yes _____   No _____
   B. If so, what are your needs and how much will it cost to meet these needs?

   Anticipated Education Needs   **Cost**

   1. _____   _____
   2. _____   _____
   3. _____   _____
   4. _____   _____
   5. _____   _____
   6. _____   _____
   7. _____   _____
   8. _____   _____
   9. _____   _____
   10. _____   _____

             Total   _____

V. Medical/Surgical Supplies
   A. Are there any medical/surgical supplies that you will need that we currently don't use?   Yes _____   No _____
   B. If so,
      1. Will we need to keep these items in stock?
                                     Yes _____   No _____
      2. How large a stock will be required? _____
      3. What specific items will you need that are not currently used?

                                           Need to Stock
           Description   **(Yes/No)**

   1. _____   _____
   2. _____   _____
   3. _____   _____
   4. _____   _____
   5. _____   _____
   6. _____   _____
   7. _____   _____
   8. _____   _____
   9. _____   _____
   10. _____   _____

VI. Charge Items/CDM
   A. When cardiac services is up and running, will the charge
      master need to be updated for new charges that are not
      currently on the charge master?   Yes _____   No _____
   B. What are the new charges and what is the current market rate?
      (Charge masters from other facilities will be available to help
      you with this task.)

      Charge Description   **Rate**

      1. _____   _____
      2. _____   _____
      3. _____   _____
      4. _____   _____
      5. _____   _____
      6. _____   _____
      7. _____   _____
      8. _____   _____
      9. _____   _____
     10. _____   _____

   C. Will your department charge tickets need to be
      changed/updated?   Yes _____   No _____
   D. Will the next order of charge tickets reflect these changes?
                                           Yes _____   No _____
   E. When will the updated charge tickets need to be ordered?
      _____ (Date)   _____ on hand? (Date)
   F. Has MIS been informed of the changes needed to order entry
      screens?   Yes _____   No _____

VII. Management Information Systems Requirements
   A. Will the implementation of CVS in your area require additional
      MIS capabilities and/or upgrades?   Yes _____   No _____
   B. If so,
      1. Is MIS aware of the impact CVS will have on your area?
                                           Yes _____   No _____
      2. What are the MIS implications in your area? (Prioritize if
         possible and be sure to include any equipment, software, or
         human resource needs.)

         _____
         _____
         _____
         _____
         _____
         _____

VIII. Policies and Procedures
- A. Will any policies and procedures related to your department need to be updated, changed, or reviewed in order to accommodate the addition of CVS? Yes _____ No _____
- B. What are they?

_____
_____
_____
_____
_____

IX. Quality Assurance
- A. What are the quality assurance issues that need to be addressed prior to the operation of CVS?

_____
_____
_____
_____

- B. What are the JCAHO requirements, if any, that your department will have to act on prior to the opening of the CVS program?

_____
_____
_____
_____

- C. What, if any, state regulations will affect the CVS project? What actions are required?

_____
_____
_____
_____

X. Other: If you have any other concerns and/or comments, please indicate below.

_____
_____
_____
_____
_____

Prepared by: _____   Date: _____

Appendix D

Cardiovascular Services Strategic Marketing Plan Outline

I. Executive Summary
II. Introduction and Background
   A. Introduction
   B. The Market Planning Process
   C. Background
III. Mission and Goals
   A. Mission Statement and Purpose
   B. Goals
IV. The Market
   A. Market Summary
   B. The Market and Its Needs
      1. Identification of major markets and their needs
      2. Target market needs
V. Life Cycle Concepts and Strategies
   A. Life Cycle Concepts
   B. Organization versus Marketplace Life Cycles
   C. The Differentiation Strategy
VI. Positioning Strategy
   A. Positioning Concepts
   B. Key Questions
   C. Positioning Strategies
   D. Summary and Conclusions
VII. Marketing Objectives
VIII. Marketing Strategies
   A. Service Strategies
   B. Physical Distribution Strategies
   C. Pricing Strategies
   D. Promotion Strategies

IX. Organization and Staffing
X. Marketing Budget
XI. Implementation Plan
XII. Evaluation and Feedback
XIII. Appendixes

Appendix E

Cardiovascular Institute Business Plan Outline

I. Executive Summary
   A. Description of Institute
   B. Statement of Mission and Role
   C. Description of Institute Programs and Services
      1. Proposed programs and services
      2. Phased implementation of programs and services
   D. Position Analysis
      1. Opportunities and threats within the market(s)
      2. Distinctive characteristics of institute programs and services
   E. Description of Equipment and Facilities
   F. Significant Technologies Involved
   G. Projected Sources and Uses of Funds
   H. Implementation Plan and Schedule
II. Marketing Analysis and Marketing Plan
   A. Description of Institute Programs and Services
      1. Public relations
      2. Fund-raising
      3. Research (basic, clinical, administrative)
      4. Education
         a. Public
         b. Professional
      5. Screening and early detection services
      6. Clinical services
      7. Community services (referral, second opinion, etc.)
      8. Statistical compilation and analysis
      9. Other/miscellaneous

B. General Description of Health Care Industry
   1. Industry trends and assumptions
   2. Cardiovascular trends and assumptions
C. Target Market Profiles and Description (by program/service, geographic market area, etc.)
   1. Consumer market(s) identification, size, trends
      a. Market, submarket identification
      b. Population and demographic analysis
      c. Profiles and trends
      d. Results of primary market research (as required)
      e. Applicable program/service identification—as user (PR, fund-raising, research, education, screening, clinical services, community services)
   2. Physician market(s) identification, size, trends
      a. Market, submarket identification
      b. Location(s) and numbers
      c. Profiles and trends
      d. Results of primary market research (as required)
      e. Applicable program/service identification—as provider, user, owner, manager (PR, fund-raising, research, education, screening, clinical services)
   3. Business/industry market(s) identification, size, trends
      a. Market, submarket identification
      b. Profiles and trends
      c. Results of primary market research (as required)
      d. Applicable program/service identification—as user, insurer/payer, cosponsor, etc. (PR, fund-raising, research, education, screening, clinical services, community services)
   4. Insurance and third-party payer market(s) identification, size, trends
      a. Market, submarket identification
      b. Managed care contracting
      c. Profiles and trends
      d. Results of primary market research (as required)
      e. Applicable program/service identification—as insurer/payer, cosponsor (PR, education, screening, clinical services, community services)
   5. Other market(s) identification, size, trends
D. Competitor Analysis (Existing and Potential)
   1. Institute/hospital competitor(s)
      a. Name, location, affiliation
      b. Program and service offered, distinguishing characteristics
      c. Pricing/contracting considerations
      d. Key physician components

     2. Allied physician/medical group competitors
       a. Names, locations
       b. Institute/hospital affiliation(s)
       c. Medical group, managed care contracting organization affiliations/alliances
       d. Distinguishing characteristics
       e. Contracting considerations
     3. Other competitors (as identified)
  E. Demand Forecasts/Projected Utilization (hospital and/or institute, depending on site, organizational structure, centralization/decentralization of services, etc.)
     1. Clinical services
       a. Cardiology (invasive/noninvasive)
       b. Cardiovascular surgery
       c. Rehabilitation
       d. Ancillary and support services
     2. Education
       a. Public
       b. Professional
     3. Screening, early detection programs
     4. Community services
  F. Marketing mix analysis (the consumer's motivation to utilize)
     1. Product/service
       a. Consumer needs and service offering
       b. Quality issues
     2. Pricing
       a. Pricing strategies
       b. Packaging strategies
       c. Pricing versus cost
     3. Place/service delivery
       a. Location(s) — clinical services, education, screening, etc.
       b. Marketing considerations of site(s) locations
       c. Delivery mechanisms (hours of operation, scheduling, physician referral systems, community referrals, etc.)
     4. Promotion/sales
       a. Promotional activities
       b. Sales plan (as appropriate)
       c. Advertising and media selection
III. Human Resources Plan
  A. Management Team
     1. Description of key personnel
     2. Team background and experience
  B. Management Staff Requirements
  C. Personnel Requirements (by site, program/service, etc.)

D. Affiliated Physician Requirements (medical directors, screening program physicians, research associates, etc.)
E. Recruitment/Retention Strategy for Required Nursing and Other Skilled Personnel in Short Supply

IV. Operations Analysis and Plan
A. Geographic Location(s) — Institute
B. Organization
   1. Legal structure — institute, other clinical/research components, by site or other variable (e.g. joint venture, partnership, etc.)
   2. Management organization chart
   3. Board of directors composition and role
   4. Relationship to other organizations (hospital, corporate, corporate members, etc.)
   5. Insurance considerations
   6. Other organizational considerations
C. Facilities
   1. Physical plant description
     a. Administrative/supportive
     b. Clinical
     c. Educational
     d. Research
     e. Other/miscellaneous
   2. Relationship to hospital(s) facilities
   3. Technology assessment
   4. Capital equipment requirements
     a. Administrative/support
     b. Clinical
     c. Educational
     d. Research
     e. Other/miscellaneous
   5. Timetable and implementation
D. Services
   1. Patient diagnostic and treatment
   2. Research
   3. Marketing
   4. Practice management
   5. Fund-raising
   6. Medical education
   7. Community education
   8. Other
E. Hours of Operation/Scheduling
F. Patient/Physician Referral Systems
G. Timetable for Implementation
H. Critical Risks and Potential Problems

V. Financial Plan
   A. Business Financial Strategies
      1. Revenue enhancement
      2. Program and service development criteria
      3. Technology procurement
      4. Physician recruitment and development
      5. Nurse recruitment and retention
      6. Other financial strategies
   B. Profit/Loss Statements for Three Years (with assumptions)
   C. Cash Flow for Three Years
   D. Budgets for Three Years (with assumptions)
   E. Financial Reporting Mechanisms
   F. Other
VI. Appendixes

Glossary

Ablation: Removal of tissue; in electrophysiology: removal or destruction of dysfunctional cardiac conduction tissue by high-energy electric current delivered via a catheter.

Ambulatory EKG recording: *See* **Holter monitor.**

Angina pectoris: Chest pain; a condition resulting from reduced blood supply to cardiac muscle tissue.

Angiography: Radiographic (X-ray) imaging and filming of the circulatory system and/or cardiac structures.

Angioplasty: Catheterization procedure to widen narrowed arteries by means of a fluid-filled, balloon-tipped catheter, which is inflated to reduce the arterial narrowing.

Arrhythmia (dysrhythmia): Abnormal cardiac rhythm; several different abnormalities including rapid heart rate (tachycardia), slow heart rate (bradycardia), cardiac rhythm originating in abnormal regions of the heart's conduction system (ventricular tachycardia, junctional rhythms), and abnormal cardiac rhythms originating above the ventricular level (supraventricular arrhythmias).

Arteriosclerosis (atherosclerosis): Vascular disease process manifested by fat, cholesterol, and other deposits within arterial walls causing narrowing of the blood flow channel (lumen) of the artery. These deposits are known as plaque.

Atherectomy: Catheterization procedure to remove arterial plaque.

Automatic implantable cardioverter/defibrillator (AICD): Implantation device that monitors cardiac rhythm. When life-threatening arrhythmia is present, the AICD delivers an electrical shock to the heart to reestablish normal cardiac rhythm.

Balloon angioplasty: *See* **Percutaneous transluminal coronary angioplasty (PTCA).**

Balloon catheter: Balloon-tipped catheter that is guided into place within a narrowed artery and inflated to widen the narrowed segment.

Biplane catheterization: Radiographic (X-ray) technique using two planes of X-ray imaging. This allows filming of two views of the same structure (for example, artery, cardiac chamber) simultaneously. Biplane technique reduces the contrast media (dye) necessary to perform a complete angiogram. *See* **Single-plane catheterization.**

C-arm radiography: Radiographic equipment design that allows the X-ray imaging system to move and rotate around the patient.

Cardiac arrest: Cessation of cardiac contraction; lack of heartbeat.

Cardiac gating: Technique using the patient's EKG signal to time and activate imaging sequences of the heart.

Cardiac ischemia: Reduced blood flow to the heart.

Cardiac output computer: Device used to estimate the amount of blood being circulated by a heart; computers may operate on thermal or dye dilution methods.

Cardiac perfusion: Flow of nutrients and oxygenated blood to the heart muscle.

Cardiomyopathy: Disease of the heart muscle.

Catheter ablation: Therapeutic application of electrophysiology (EP) that causes tissue to lose its ability to conduct electrical signals.

Catheterization: Invasive technique of examining the heart and circulatory system by inserting a small tube (catheter) into an artery or vein.

Cineangiography: Radiographic (X-ray) technique using high-speed filming of the circulatory system and/or cardiac structures.

Cine computed tomography (CT): Diagnostic modality for coronary artery disease; currently under research (along with cine magnetic resonance imaging — cine MRI — as possible replacement for coronary angiography; operates at high speed (approximately 25 images per second).

Cine magnetic resonance imaging (cine MRI): *See* **Cine computed tomography (CT).**

Congestive heart failure: Condition resulting from the heart's inability to pump all of the blood returning from the venous system.

Continuous wave Doppler: Diagnostic evaluation of blood flow velocity and volume to assess narrowing of the cardiac valve opening.

Contrast media: Iodine-based dye used to image the circulatory system and/or heart.

Coronary arteries: The two arteries that provide the blood supply to the heart muscle.

Coronary artery bypass graft (CABG): Surgical procedure to improve the blood supply to the heart muscle. Involves routing the heart muscle blood supply past narrowings in the patient's coronary arteries by using vein grafts or redirecting another artery within the chest (internal mammary artery).

Coronary artery disease: Condition resulting from insufficient blood supply to the heart muscle.

Coronary occlusion: Obstruction, either partial or complete, of a coronary artery resulting in reduced or blocked blood supply to the segment of cardiac muscle (myocardium) being fed by the artery.

Cryoablation: Diagnostic electrophysiology (EP) procedure to freeze injured heart tissue.

Cyanosis: Duskiness or bluish tinge of the skin caused by reduced oxygen content of the blood.

Defibrillator: Device used to shock the heart muscle when severe arrhythmias have been detected, thus allowing the heart to reestablish a normal rhythm.

Digital subtraction angiography: Use of an imaging computer system to "subtract" the artifact in an angiographic image to produce an enhanced picture.

Dissection: Abnormal splitting of a vessel wall that may result in an occlusion; a complication of angioplasty procedures.

Doppler: Ultrasound technique that utilizes reflected sound energy to determine the direction and velocity of blood flow.

Dysrhythmia: *See* **Arrhythmia.**

Echocardiography: Cardiac ultrasound imaging; noninvasive diagnostic procedure to visualize cardiac wall motion and valve function and to test for structural abnormalities for congenital heart disease. Also called cardiac ultrasound/Doppler, echo/Doppler, cardiac/Doppler.

Echo Doppler: Ultrasound technology used to evaluate blood-flow direction and velocity.

Ejection fraction: Mathematical computation of the heart's contraction capability.

Electrocardiography: Procedure for recording and studying electrical signals originating from the heart; the graphic records of signals are called electrocardiograms.

Electrophysiology: Invasive diagnosis and treatment of cardiac conduction disorders.

Endothelium: Inner lining of numerous anatomical structures, including the heart and blood vessels.

Excimer laser: Cool laser energy.

Extracorporeal cardiopulmonary support: Heart–lung bypass pump.

Extracorporeal perfusion: Use of heart–lung pump to supply oxygenated blood to a patient during cardiac surgery.

Fluoroscopy: "Live" radiographic (X-ray) imaging of body structures. Used in cardiac catheterization to visualize the catheter path so as to position it correctly for contrast injections or for angioplasty procedures.

Gated blood pool study: Nuclear cardiographic procedure that uses the patient's EKG signal to trigger imaging sequences of the heart to evaluate the cardiac contraction patterns (ejection fraction).

Hemodynamic monitoring: Recording and evaluation of intravascular pressures during cardiac catheterization.

Holter monitor: Device that measures cardiac rhythm (EKCG signal) during exercise to allow for computer scanning over a 24-hour period. Also called ambulatory EKG recording.

Image intensifier: Component of the radiographic (X-ray) system that generates the image of the structure(s) being visualized for both the video system and the filming system; a critical element of a cardiac catheterization laboratory.

Interventional cardiology: Term used to describe therapeutic invasive cardiology procedure (for example, PTCA, atherectomy, valvuloplasty).

Intra-aortic balloon pump (IABP): Device used to assist blood circulation by reducing the work load required to pump blood to the body. The balloon system is inserted into the femoral artery and placed in the aorta, where it is controlled by a pumping system being triggered from an EKG signal.

Invasive cardiology: Cardiology procedures that require the insertion of devices into the body; cardiac catheterization is an invasive cardiology procedure.

Ischemic heart disease (myocardial ischemia): Condition resulting from narrowed coronary arteries, which restrict the flow of blood to the heart muscle.

Left ventricular assist device (LVAD): Artificial implantable or external pumping device used to reduce amount of injury to the heart due to myocardial infarction, valvular infection, or valvular dysfunction or to support the patient's circulatory capacity on a temporary basis. *See* **Intra-aortic balloon pump (IABP).**

Lipoprotein (LDL, HDL): Substance composed of lipid and protein. Low-density lipoprotein (LDL) is considered to be the harmful carrier of cholesterol in blood; high-density lipoprotein (HDL) is considered to be beneficial because it is thought to carry cholesterol from the tissue to be metabolized and removed from the body.

Lumen: The inner opening of a tube, as in a blood vessel or a catheter.

Mitral valve prolapse: Abnormal bowing of the mitral valve leaflet(s) during ventricular contraction.

MuGA study: Multiple-gated acquisition; nuclear cardiographic procedure that utilizes the patient's EKG rhythm to time cardiac imaging sequences.

Myocardial infarction: Damage or death of myocardial tissue (heart muscle) due to reduced blood supply.

Myocardial perfusion: Flow of oxygenated blood to and through the heart muscle.

Myocardium: Heart muscle tissue.

Noninvasive cardiology: Diagnostic cardiology procedures that require either no penetration or minimal penetration of the skin; electrocardiography and echocardiography are examples of noninvasive procedures.

Nuclear cardiography: Diagnostic cardiology procedures that use injected radionucleide material for imaging.

Oximeter: A device that determines the oxygen saturation levels of blood; used extensively in cardiac catheterization laboratories.

Pacemaker: The region of the heart that generates the electrical signal to cause cardiac contraction (sinoatrial, or SA, node); an artificial pacemaker (permanent pacemaker implant or PPI) controls cardiac rhythm through the use of a battery-powered generator unit and wires, which are placed in contact with the heart muscle tissue.

Percutaneous transluminal coronary angioplasty (PTCA): Balloon angioplasty procedure that involves directing a balloon-tipped catheter through the skin to a plaque-blocked coronary artery via a larger catheter, known as a guiding catheter, and over a small placement wire, known as a guide wire. After correct placement of the fluid-filled balloon, the physician inflates it to widen the blocked area of the coronary artery lumen so that the blood supply to the heart muscle is reinstated.

Perfusion pump: Heart–lung machine.

Pericarditis: Inflammation of the sac (pericardium) that surrounds the heart.

Physiologic monitoring: Electronic display and recording device used to observe and record multiple physiologic parameters (for example, EKG signal, arterial blood pressure, blood pressure within cardiac chambers). This unit is an integral part of the cardiac catheterization laboratory.

Positron emission tomography (PET): A diagnostic technology used to evaluate metabolic processes within the body.

Pulsed wave Doppler: Noninvasive diagnostic procedure to detect evidence of abnormal flow due to narrowing of cardiac valve opening.

Reperfusion therapy: Recently developed technique that allows delivery of oxygenated blood to myocardial tissue that has had its normal channel of blood flow obstructed. The process involves forcing oxygenated blood retrograde (backward) through the coronary sinus (cardiac vein) to reach the compromised tissue.

Sensitometry: Cine film (heart cath film) quality control procedure to assess the function of the film-processing system (cine film processor). Associated with densitometry evaluation process, which allows evaluation of the radiographic (X-ray) filming system.

Septal defect: Abnormal opening between two chambers of the heart occurring in one or both of the walls that separate the cardiac chambers; atrial septal defect (ASD) or ventricular septal defect (VSD).

Single-photon emission computerized tomography (SPECT): Improved nuclear cardiographic procedure that enhances imaging resolution and reduces imaging times.

Single-plane catheterization: Radiographic (X-ray) system that uses one plane, or view, of imaging as opposed to biplane or two simultaneous imaging views.

Sinus rhythm: Normal heart rhythm; originates in the sinus node, an area of specialized nerve cells that acts as a natural pacemaker of the heart.

Steerable catheter: Angioplasty catheter and guide-wire system that affords enhanced positioning capabilities within the coronary arteries during surgery.

Stenosis: Abnormal narrowing of area of tissue, such as a cardiac valve or the lumen of a coronary artery.

Streptokinase: Blood clot–dissolving drug used to reopen a blocked artery.

Swan–Ganz catheterization: Use of a right-heart catheter to measure intravascular pressures from the right-heart chambers and the pulmonary arteries.

With its large balloon tip, the catheter can be wedged into smaller pulmonary capillaries to measure approximate pressure from the left atrium. May also be used to perform thermodilution cardiac output and to infuse medications into the patient's central venous system.

Thallium study: Nuclear cardiographic procedure that utilizes the radionuclide thallium, an isotope that will tag itself to normally oxygenated heart muscle tissue to assist in the detection of coronary artery disease.

Thermal laser: Heat laser energy with addition of metal cap ("hot tip").

Thrombolytic agents: Pharmaceuticals used to dissolve, or lyse, blood clots.

Thrombus: Blood clot that has formed in a blood vessel or cardiac chamber; plural *thrombi.*

t-PA (tissue plasminogen activator): Thrombolytic drug used to dissolve blood clots of recent formation in the coronary arteries.

Transesophageal echo/Doppler (TEE): Variation of ultrasound procedure during which a transducer is mounted on the tip of an esophageal probe and inserted into the esophagus to yield images of the heart taken in close proximity to cardiac structures and to allow blood flow recordings.

Transvenous defibrillator: Recently developed device implanted much like an artificial pacemaker, but it performs like an automatic implantable cardioverter/defibrillator. The monitoring and energy delivering leads are implanted transvenously.

Triglyceride: Normal chemical form in which most fats exist in the body.

Ultrasound: High-frequency sound used noninvasively to image organs within the body.

Ultrasound transducer: Ultrasound generator–receiver unit that helps technologist transmit and receive energy from the heart so as to generate an echocardiograph.

Urokinase: Thrombolytic, blood clot–dissolving enzyme derived from human urine.

Valvular commissurotomy: Surgical repair for insufficient (leaky) valve.

Valvuloplasty: Invasive procedure to enlarge constricted cardiac valves.

Vascular stent insertion: Insertion of a device that is delivered to the site within an artery to minimize narrowing or obstruction.

Vectorcardiography: Process of measuring and recording the electrical energy vectors that originate in and through the heart muscle.

Ventriculogram: Radiographic image of the ventricle (generally the left), recorded on film during cardiac catheterization.

Video freeze frame: The capability during cardiac catheterization, mainly PTCA procedures, to stop the playback of a recorded video image at a specific point to demonstrate the pathology of interest.

Video road mapping: A process that, when used during PTCA procedures, allows the physician to orient to the area of coronary artery stenosis by referencing the "frozen" image showing the narrowed region and the live image while directing the angioplasty catheter into position.